FIRST EDITION

ISBN 978-1-7775152-4-9 (print)

ISBN 978-1-7775152-5-6 (eBook)

www.dryoumethod.com

Instagram: @dr.you.official

Declaration

No funding was received from any source to write this book or recommend any resource. Aside from my own book *Fire Anatomy Mnemonics*, I do not make any profit from any of the recommendations in this book. **Any recommendations I make are because I genuinely believe they are excellent resources.**

There are also no affiliate marketing links. Any video or website links provided are simply for your convenience.

Accessing Video and Website Links

Video and website links appear throughout this book, especially in the *Subjects* section. If using the eBook version of this book, you can simply click on the links to open them. If using the print version, all the links are compiled and sorted neatly on the following page for your convenience:

www.dryoumethod.com/companion_links

Simply bookmark this page and refer to it as needed.

Acknowledgements

Many thanks to my editor, Paul Mayhew, for his outstanding commitment, professionalism and genuine helpfulness.

Preface

What is this book?

Medical school is a gargantuan challenge, and as a wee new medical student, it was really intimidating on a number of levels. The pace was tenacious. Students were failing or dropping out like flies. I was stressed that any given test could be the one that ruins me. I wasn't sure if I'd have a life for the next four years or if I'd be miserable all throughout. I clearly remember thinking, "What did I get myself into...?!"

I was also confused about a lot of things, and by the looks of it, many of my peers were as well. It took me a long time to grasp what standardized exams I needed to take and when to take them. It also wasn't clear what the optimal approach to studying for each subject was and what resources to use (of which there were so many!) Everyone had their own approach and gave different recommendations, some of which were questionable. As a result, a lot of the basic sciences was trial and error, and if I were to go back and do it again, I'd do a lot of things differently.

In my final year of medical school - having hindsight of all the things that worked well and those that didn't – I wrote this book to serve as a super-concise yet comprehensive companion for students in the basic science years.

Fire Medical School Companion is not meant to replicate *First Aid for the USMLE Step 1*, a book I strongly recommend every student uses. *First Aid* presents all high-yield information for almost all major basic science topics and diseases; this book, on the other hand, teaches you how to approach each subject, offers optimal strategies to use, and provides unique mnemonics and tricks. In effect, this book is ideally used in tandem with *First Aid* and I have tried to avoid repeating things, such as mnemonics, that are in *First Aid*, to keep your studies as efficient as possible.

This book also contains unique sections addressing matters of lifestyle, motivation and mental health, and study strategies for the basic sciences.

It's my sincere wish that this guide makes your medical school life significantly easier and more enjoyable. Have a great time reading!

Dr. Yousuf Saqib

March 2022

Contents

Lab Values

SI and conventional units are essentially like metric and imperial units for lab values. Most of the world uses SI units, while the US uses conventional units.

➤ **Blood, Plasma, Serum**	SI	Conventional
Alanine aminotransferase (ALT)	8–20 U/L	
Aspartate aminotransferase (AST)	8–20 U/L	
Amylase, serum	25–125 U/L	
Bilirubin, direct	0–5 µmol/L	0.0–0.3 mg/dL
Bilirubin, total	2–17 µmol/L	0.1–1.0 mg/dL
Calcium (Total)	2.1–2.8 mmol/L	8.4–10.2 mg/dL
Cholesterol (Total)	< 5.2 mmol/L	< 200 mg/dL
Creatinine, serum (Total)	53–106 µmol/L	0.6–1.2 mg/dL
Electrolytes, serum		
Sodium	136–145 (mmol/L & mEq/L)	
Chloride	95–105 (mmol/L & mEq/L)	
Potassium	3.5–5.0 (mmol/L & mEq/L)	
Bicarbonate	22–28 (mmol/L & mEq/L)	
Magnesium	0.75–1.0 mmol/L	1.5 mEq/L
Gases, arterial blood (room air)		
PO2	75–105 mm Hg	
PCO2	33–44 mm Hg	
pH	7.35–7.45	
Glucose, serum (Fasting)	3.8–6.1 mmol/L	70–110 mg/dL
2-h postprandial	< 6.6 mmol/L	< 120 mg/dL
Growth hormone – arginine stimulation (Fasting)	< 5 (µg/L & ng/mL)	
Osmolality, serum	275–295 mOsm/kg	
Phosphatase (alkaline), serum	20–70 U/L	
Phosphorus (inorganic), serum	1.0–1.5 mmol/L	3.0–4.5 mg/dL
Prolactin, serum (hPRL)	< 20 (µg/L & ng/mL)	
Proteins, serum		
Total (recumbent)	60–78 g/L	6.0–7.8 g/dL
Albumin	35–55 g/L	3.5–5.5 g/dL
Globulins	23–35 g/L	2.3–3.5 g/dL
Urea nitrogen, serum (BUN)	1.2–3.0 mmol/L	7–18 mg/dL
Uric acid, serum	0.18–0.48 mmol/L	3.0–8.2 mg/dL

Cerebrospinal Fluid	SI	Conventional
Cell count	0–5 (x10^6/L & /mm^3)	
Glucose	2.2–3.9 mmol/L	40–70 mg/dL
Proteins	< 0.40 g/L	< 40 mg/dL

Hematologic	SI	Conventional
Erythrocyte count	Male: 4.3–5.9 (×10^{12}/L & million/mm^3) Female: 3.5–5.5 (×10^{12}/L & million/mm^3)	
Erythrocyte sedimentation rate (ESR)	Male: 0–15 mm/h Female: 0–20 mm/h	
Hematocrit (Hct)	Male: 0.41–0.53 Female: 0.36–0.46	41–53% 36–46%
Hemoglobin (Hb)	Male: 135–175 g/L Female: 120–160 g/L	13.5–17.5 g/dL 12.0–16.0 g/dL

Leukocyte count and differential
  Leukocytes, total
    Neutrophils
    Lymphocytes
    Monocytes
    Eosinophils
    Basophils
	
	4.5–11.0 × 10^9/L
	0.54–0.62
	0.25–0.33
	0.03–0.05
	0.01–0.03
	0–0.0075
		
		4500–11,000/mm^3
		54–62%
		25–33%
		3–7%
		1–3%
		0–0.75%

Mean corpuscular hemoglobin	25.4–34.6 pg/cell	
Mean corpuscular volume	80–100 (fL & μm^3)	

Coagulation
  Prothrombin time (PT)
  Partial thromboplastin time (aPTT)
	
	11–15 seconds
	25–40 seconds	

Platelet count	150–400 × 10^9/L	150,000–400,000/mm^3
Reticulocyte count	0.005–0.015	0.5–1.5%

Sweat	SI	Conventional
Chloride	0–35 mmol/L	

Urine	SI	Conventional
Proteins, total	< 0.15 g/24 h	< 150 mg/24 h

*Values may vary from lab to lab and regionally

How to use this book

Early, new, or forthcoming students

If you're looking for comprehensive help for medical school, consider reading *Sections 1-5* from start to finish, like you would a regular book. Then, when you start learning a particular subject in school (e.g., anatomy), read that subject's chapter in *Section 6*.

Experienced students reviewing for standardized exams

If you're an experienced student simply looking to enhance your review for particular subjects, skim through the *table of contents* to see if there's anything in *Sections 1-5* that interests you. If not, proceed straight to your subject of interest's chapter in *Section 6*.

SECTION 1

Medical School Overview

If you haven't got a clue what each stage of your medical journey looks like, what standardized exams you'll need to take, when to start preparing, etc., *relax* – you're not the only one who's confused. The medical journey is daunting, and it takes quite a while to grasp its nuances.

This section outlines the *most important* details for you to know about your medical journey. Specific details are mentioned for those aiming to obtain a residency position in the US, UK, or Canada.

> ## ➤ 1. Stages of the medical journey

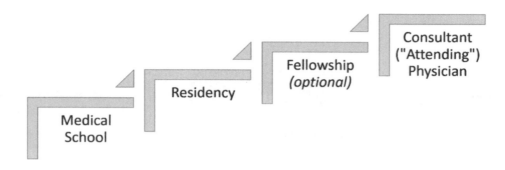

Medical School

Medical school is where you learn the basic "bread and butter" of medical knowledge and skills. You learn about all the major diseases, medications, and basic history-taking and physical exam skills.

By the time you graduate, you should be able to work alongside an attending physician in any specialty, and have a reasonable idea of how to manage the patients in a very general sense. You *WON'T* be expected to know the doses for most medications, perform advanced procedures, or manage patients entirely on your own – these are mastered later, in residency.

Residency

Residency is where you learn to become an independently practicing physician in the specialty you've chosen. Although you're officially a doctor upon graduation from medical school, all doctors must complete a residency program to actually be able to practice *on their own*.

Residency is an actual job, and you rightly get paid for it, though much less than a consultant physician's salary. For example, if an attending physician in your specialty makes $300,000 a year, a first-year resident might make around $60,000. Residencies are generally 2 to 5 years in length, with primary care specialties on the shorter side and most surgical specialties being around five years. A few specialties, like neurosurgery, may reach up to 7 years in length.

Here are typical lengths of residency programs for different specialties in the US and Canada in 2022:

Specialty	US	Canada
Anesthesiology	3 years + a transitional year	5 years
Cardiac Surgery	6 years	6 years
Cardiology	3 years Internal Medicine + 3 years Cardiology fellowship	3 years Internal Medicine + 3 years Cardiology fellowship
Dermatology	3 years + a transitional year	5 years
Emergency Medicine	3-4 years	5 years
Family Practice	3 years	2 years
General Surgery	5 years	5 years
Internal Medicine	3 years	3-4 years
Neurology	3 years + a transitional year	5 years
Neurosurgery	6-7 years	6 years
Obstetrics/Gynecology	4 years	5 years
Ophthalmology	3 years + a transitional year	5 years
Orthopedic Surgery	5 years	5 years
Otolaryngology (Head & Neck Surgery)	5 years	5 years
Pathology	4 years	4 years (Hematological) or 5 years (Anatomical, General, Neuropathology)
Pediatrics	3 years	4 years
Physical Medicine	3-4 years	5 years
Plastic Surgery	5-6 years	5 years
Psychiatry	4 years	5 years
Public Health	3 years	5 years
Radiation Oncology	4 years + a transitional year	5 years
Radiology, Diagnostic	4 years + a transitional year	5 years
Urology	5 years	5 years
Vascular Surgery	5 years	5 years

Fellowship

A fellowship is an optional program some choose to do after their residency, where they get even more specialized training. For example, to become a trauma surgeon in Canada or the US, you must complete a general surgery residency (5 years) and then a 1–2-year fellowship in trauma surgery.

As with residencies, a fellowship is a paid job; slightly better pay than a final-year resident but still a lot less than an attending physician.

Consultant Physician

A consultant (also called an *attending*) physician is a physician who has completed their residency and is now practicing independently in their specialty. Consultants supervise fellows, residents, and medical students. They get those big doctor salaries you like looking up on Google.

> 2. Stages of medical school

Medical school can generally be divided into two phases: **basic science years** and **clinical years**.

Basic Science Years

Your basic science years are essentially where you learn basic medical principles and facts, primarily from textbooks and lectures. Your focus is mainly on understanding how the body works and what the various diseases are, rather than the nuances of diagnosis and treatment. In a four-year program, your basic sciences are usually your first two years and usually include:

- Clinical skills
- Anatomy
- Embryology
- Histology
- Ethics
- Epidemiology and Biostatistics
- Biochemistry
- Genetics
- Microbiology
- Immunology
- Psychiatry
- Physiology
- Pharmacology
- Pathology

Clinical Years

After your basic science years come your clinical years, when you will work and learn in hospitals and clinics. This is when you learn a lot more about the practical aspects of caring for patients, like diagnostic criteria and treatment protocols. You will:

- see real patients, take their history, and examine them;
- present your findings to your consultant physicians, often on ward rounds (the visiting of patients on the ward by the entire team every morning);
- get to observe and often participate in diagnostic and therapeutic procedures (e.g., surgeries in your surgery rotation).

In a four-year program, these are your final two years.

Clinical rotations can be divided into **core rotations** and **elective rotations**.

Core rotations

These are mandatory rotations that every student must complete. Most schools have five or six core rotations, usually including (in no particular order):

- Internal medicine – 12 weeks
- Surgery – 12 weeks
- Psychiatry – 6 weeks
- Pediatrics – 6 weeks
- Obstetrics/gynecology – 6 weeks
- Family medicine (some schools) – 6 weeks

Elective rotations

These are rotations that you can do in any specialty you desire, e.g., neurosurgery, dermatology, radiology, etc. You're usually required to complete around 24–30 weeks of these. Elective rotations often come with less evaluations and course work. These are good opportunities to test out specialties to see if you'd like to pursue them, get letters of recommendation in your hopeful specialty, and build connections with staff of residency programs that you hope to apply to.

> ➤ **3. Major standardized exams**

Out of all major standardized examinations for the US, UK, and Canada, **the United States Medical Licensure Examination (USMLE) Step 1 is the only one for the basic sciences** (vs. all other exams mentioned below, which are taken during or after clinical years and focus on *clinical* medicine). This exam is not required for UK or Canadian programs. Therefore, if you're planning on applying only to UK or Canadian residency programs, you don't have to worry about taking any major standardized exams until your clinical years.

The **Canadian NAC exam** and the **UK PLAB test** are the only two major exams required exclusively for international medical graduates (IMGs) to be able to apply for residency programs in those countries, i.e., native Canadian/UK applicants don't need to do them.

The rest of the following exams are required by all (IMG and native) to apply for residency programs.

US Examinations

	USMLE Step 1	USMLE Step 2 CK (clinical knowledge)
Who must take it?	All applicants to US programs	
Timing	End of year 2 (optimally before start of clinical rotations)	After completing core rotations and before submitting residency applications (around early 4th year)
Content	All basic science knowledge	All knowledge from core rotations
Format	Multiple choice	
Duration	8 hours (Seven 1-hour blocks, with 1 hour of total break time to use as you like between blocks)	9 hours (Eight 1-hour blocks, with 1 hour of total break time to use as you like between blocks)
Scoring	Pass/Fail	Score between 1-300 (Passing score: 209)

[There used to be a USMLE Step 2 CS – a clinical skills exam – but in January of 2021 it was permanently discontinued in the wake of the COVID-19 pandemic.]

Canadian Examinations

	MCCQE Part 1	NAC Exam
Who must take it?	All applicants to Canadian programs	Only IMG applicants to Canadian programs
Timing	After completing core rotations and before submitting residency applications (around early 4th year)	
Content	All knowledge from core rotations	History-taking, physical examination, and basic knowledge of diagnostics and management
Format	Multiple choice and short answer	OSCE
Duration	8 hours (4 hours straight of multiple-choice questions, then 45-minute break, then 3.5 hours straight of short answer questions)	~2 hours 15 minutes (Ten 11-minute stations, with 2 minutes between stations)
Scoring	Score between 100-400 (Passing score: 226)	Score between 1300-1500 (Passing score: 1374)

The MCCQE Part 1 is essentially the equivalent of the USMLE Step 2 CK, and the NAC exam is essentially the equivalent of what used to be the USMLE Step 2 CS (now discontinued).

UK Examinations

	PLAB Test	Multi-Specialty Recruitment Assessment (MSRA)
Who must take it?	Only IMG applicants to UK programs	Only applicants to certain specialties*
Timing	After graduation from medical school	After submission of residency applications
Content	Part 1: All knowledge from core rotations Part 2: History-taking, physical examination, and practical skills	Professional dilemmas and clinical problem solving
Format	Part 1: Multiple choice Part 2: OSCE	Multiple choice, matching, and rank-in-order
Duration	Part 1: 3 hours Part 2: ~3 hours (sixteen 8-minute scenarios)	170 minutes (95 minutes for Professional Dilemmas paper; 75 minutes for Clinical Problem-Solving paper)
Scoring	Pass/Fail	Numerical score (variable)

Specialties that require MSRA: general practice (family medicine), anesthetics, psychiatry (core and CAMHS), emergency medicine, radiology, ophthalmology, neurosurgery, obstetrics and gynecology, community and sexual reproductive health, and pediatrics.

The PLAB Part 1 is essentially the equivalent of the USMLE Step 2 CK (albeit much shorter), and the PLAB Part 2 is essentially the equivalent of what used to be the USMLE Step 2 CS (now discontinued), plus some practical skills (e.g., venipuncture, urinary catheterization, etc.)

➤ 4. Residency applications

Residency Applications for US, Canada, and UK

	US	Canada	UK
Application Portal	ERAS	CaRMS	Oriel
When Applications Open	September	October	November
Residency Start Date	June (of following year)	July (of following year)	August (of following year)

Start thinking of your residency preference during your core rotations

It's useful to have a rough idea of which specialties you would like to consider while you're in your core rotations, so that you can plan elective rotations in those specialties. This is important so that you can gain first-hand experience of a specialty to really know if it is for you or not. Keep in mind that a key part of your residency application is having completed an elective in the specialty and having letters of recommendation from consultants in it.

It is also, of course, fine to be thinking about residency specialties during your basic sciences. This can be great to dream about and provide real motivation. However, just bear in mind that nothing compares to first-hand experience in a specialty during clinical rotations, so don't commit yourself entirely until you have real experience under your belt.

Have a set idea by the start of final year: residency application time!

Keep in mind many students apply to more than one specialty. In fact, this is generally the wisest choice for IMGs given the greater competition they face. If you desire, you can switch specialties more easily once you've gotten your foot in the door and completed 6-12 months of residency in the country.

When do you have to start worrying about residency applications?

Aside from completing standardized exams, there's really just one main thing you need to start preparing *before* your actual residency applications open up: **elective(s) in the specialty** and **letters of recommendation** (collected during your *clinical rotations*). The rest of your application is handled when applications open up. In other words, you do not need to be directly preparing anything for applications in your basic sciences years. Simply focus on your studies!

SECTION 2

Lifestyle and Time Management

Medical school requires a substantial amount of studying just to get by, and even more if you want to excel.

We're human beings, though, and we have to reconcile with the fact that we have meaningful needs outside of simply studying, eating, and sleeping. Therefore, the essence of this section is around building sustainable and enjoyable long-term habits that increase our productivity but minimize stress. This section also provides important guidelines and advice on matters such as financials and involvement in research.

> **1. Making studying enjoyable**

PRINCIPLE

Make studying enjoyable by:

1) **Optimizing study conditions,**
2) **Taking breaks when fatigued, and**
3) **Focusing on the intellectual challenge**

Your basic science journey is not a sprint – it's a marathon. You will almost certainly face times when you really don't feel like studying. Your job is to develop a study routine where those times are kept at a minimum. It is therefore critically important to make your studying as enjoyable as possible, such that you become conditioned to actually look forward to your study sessions.

Finding joy in studying is easier with subjects you find interesting. What's a lot more challenging is when a subject is completely unappealing to you. Rest assured, though: even in such circumstances, it is *absolutely* still possible. The following three guidelines are your foundation for doing so:

1. Optimize your study environment

Create the most pleasant conditions you can for your study environment. The material you're learning might not always be your favorite, but your *setting* can be.

Spend some time thinking about ways to make your study setting as enjoyable as possible, without it being distracting. For example, some have subconsciously grown to hate studying at home. If this is you, picture walking into a friendly, cozy coffee shop, getting your favorite hot or cold drink, finding a toasty spot by the window, and opening up your laptop for some relaxing work for a few hours. You can even play relaxing white noise on YouTube, like rain at a cabin or a warm, crackling fireplace, and chat with friends or go for a walk on your break.

Over time, this pleasant experience can condition you to really enjoy the experience of studying and to actually *look forward* to your next study session. Over the course of a few years, this adds up to an *enormous* advantage in medical school. Therefore, even if it costs you a few extra dollars per day, understand that the money you spend on making your study experience pleasant – be it on coffee, snacks, or a better study chair or desk or perhaps even headphones(!) – is an investment into your education that will pay dividends in the long run. The balance is in nurturing focus, momentum, and productive and enjoyable routines, and avoiding time-wasting, frustrations, and distractions.

Bear in mind, if you find that a study location is not working for you, change it early. Don't wait until you hit a rock bottom of motivation and productivity; once you get that feeling that "this study session is probably not going to be great", consider something as simple as changing seats. You'd be surprised how big of an impact a simple seat change can have!

Additionally, try to avoid places that you associate with leisure, like a couch you watch movies on, or the bed you sleep on. Simply sitting in those spots can bring about the urge to do those activities again. The power is in the repeated conditioning of a productive context, i.e., environment and situation.

2. Take breaks when you are tired

Minimizing mental fatigue increases studying efficiency and maintains positive associations with studying. So, when you start to feel tired, TAKE A BREAK!

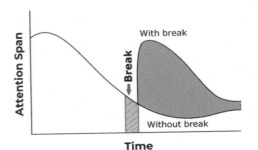

While this may seem obvious, in reality, medical students often try to "push through" fatigue, thinking this will make them more productive. But it very quickly isn't, as the mind slows and clouds, giving a depreciating return on effort.

This "pushing" also increases feelings of frustration and restlessness and contributes to negative associations with even the thought of studying. So, it is often pushing our psychology in the wrong direction! To avoid this, take a short break once you begin to feel fatigued.

Studies have shown that purposeful breaks of even 5-10 minutes can significantly increase concentration, productivity, and energy.

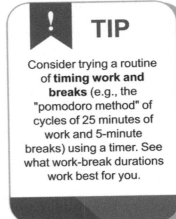

! TIP

Consider trying a routine of **timing work and breaks** (e.g., the "pomodoro method" of cycles of 25 minutes of work and 5-minute breaks) using a timer. See what work-break durations work best for you.

3. Focus on the intellectual challenge

Intelligence is not just something you're born with – it is also exercised and strengthened when you intellectually challenge yourself (and perhaps also weakens with lack of use, too!). Not only do recent studies support this,[1] simply ask any senior medical student how they feel about their problem-solving abilities now compared to *before* medical school.

Now, you might wonder what this has to do with making studying enjoyable. Think about it this

---

[1] Stankov, L., & Lee, J. (2020). We Can Boost IQ: Revisiting Kvashchev's Experiment. Journal of Intelligence, 8(4), 41.

way: every intellectual struggle or moment of confusion that you try to work through during your studying is exercising your brain and potentially providing you with lasting cognitive improvement.

Therefore, if you're not feeling particularly enthusiastic about some dry material you're learning or a subject you have little interest in, focus on the *intellectual challenge* of your task rather than just the material alone. Take pleasure in solving the puzzle in front of you and in using your intelligence to make thoughtful connections. Know that each moment of struggle is strengthening your intellectual prowess. This realization makes studying a whole lot more fun and rewarding when the material isn't on your side!

> ## ➤ 2. Study intervals

PRINCIPLE

Avoid mental fatigue by keeping the duration of your study sessions roughly between 1.5–3 hours.

As mentioned previously, once your mind becomes fatigued, efficiency decreases significantly. While some of that fatigue can be shaken off with short (5-10 minute) breaks, you will eventually reach a point where those short breaks are not enough to refresh your concentration and productivity. Ultimately, you can only study effectively for so many hours in a single session. This is your **maximum effective study duration**, after which you need to bring your session to a close.

This means it is best to avoid trying to complete your entire day's studying in one session. Instead, find the session duration that produces the best results for *you*, and remember that with time and practice your mental stamina can increase. Generally, though, this will be somewhere between **1.5 and 3 hours**, as even seasoned students will usually struggle after 3 straight hours. With that said, if sessions longer than 3 hours are still effective and enjoyable for you, go for it.

An example of a productive study day can look something like this:

MORNING 3 hours studying	BREAK (few hours)	**AFTERNOON** 2 hours studying	BREAK (few hours)	**NIGHT** 2 hours studying

➤ 3. Amount of daily study time

> **PRINCIPLE**
>
> **> 7 hours/day of *focused* studying is an excellent target, but focus more on the *results*, not the time.**

You might hear some students claiming to study absurdly high numbers of hours per day. If they report a number much greater than 9 hours per day, take it with a grain of salt. It is highly unlikely this is all focused and productive studying time. Not only is this amount of daily studying not feasible for most students, but it's also not necessary.

Think back to the ultimate purpose of studying: learning, understanding, and retaining information. Simply sitting at your desk with your book or laptop in front of you is not the aim. This is not a "clock-watching" exercise; it is about active and positive studying. Once mental fatigue sets in, efficiency and positivity drop significantly. While you might feel dedicated, hardworking, and perhaps a little pious by forcing yourself to study after this point, it becomes increasingly difficult and inefficient.

In other words, not only do you start to feel miserable, but you are likely getting very little benefit from this time and effort. At that point, your time would be better spent taking a break and coming back later, refreshed and more motivated.

Therefore, focus more on the *quality* of results (i.e., learning the very best that you can) rather the *quantity* of time. As a rough metric, however, if you can get **7 hours** of *focused*, *efficient* studying done on a class-free day, you can call that an excellent study day. If you can keep that productivity up, it is enough for most students to excel.

Note that on class days, targets are much more variable and depend on different factors, like hours spent in class, etc.

➤ 4. Leisure time

> **PRINCIPLE**
>
> **Have something to look forward to doing, every day.**

Daily

Outside of time spent eating, showering, exercising, etc., it's reasonable to have around **1-1.5 hours** of pure leisure time in your day. In this time, try to detach yourself from work and do immersive things you really enjoy, whether it's playing video games, playing or watching sports, hanging out with friends, or anything else. By doing this, you have something to look forward to enjoying even on unpleasant days when school isn't going your way. This is critical for "topping up your reserves" and your endurance as a student.

Remember: your basic science journey is a marathon – not a sprint.

One day a week

Although taking an entire day off is generally not advisable, it's perfectly reasonable to take one day a week (i.e., on the weekend) a bit easier. You can increase your leisure time on this day and do something you wouldn't normally be able to do most days, while also getting a moderate amount of work done.

For example, supposing you normally aim for 8 hours of studying on off-days. You can instead complete 4 hours in the morning and then take the rest of the day off (it being easier to get work "out of the way" in the morning than starting in the afternoon). See what works for you and be sure to consider the context. If you have several exams coming up, you'll have to work a bit harder, but you can have some catch-up time off afterwards.

After an exam

After you complete a major exam or set of exams, and you don't have any others in the near future, it's important to reward yourself. It's therefore not unreasonable to take the rest of that day completely off if you like (see *Rewards After Exams,* below).

> **5. Rewards after exams**

PRINCIPLE
Condition yourself, through rewards, to love that post-exam feeling.

Just as we discussed above the importance of creating positive associations with the action of studying, it's also very fruitful for your long-term medical school endurance to create similar positive associations with your exams.

Rewards after exams are a powerful source of motivation. They're especially valuable because the harder you work, the better the reward tends to feel. For a vivid example, think about fasting. After working hard the entire day and avoiding food and drink, that first sip of water – a substance you normally drink all throughout the day without much thought or excitement – can feel so sublime that you look forward to that feeling again and again.

Similarly, by rewarding yourself with something you really enjoy after a major exam or set of exams, especially when you've worked hard, that post-exam feeling can be utterly uplifting. These fond experiences and associations stick with you and serve as a powerful motivator to work even harder. In the long run, this can truly make the difference between a gloomy, low-spirited medical school experience and a rewarding, exciting one.

Keep in mind, however, that one of the most potent rewards is the satisfaction of knowing you did well on an exam. So, work hard to try to achieve that, as it creates a positive feedback loop (work hard → great results → motivation to work harder, etc.). However, results are not always in your control, and sometimes things don't turn out in your favor, but if you can get them to be favorable, more often than not, you're on the right track!

➤ 6. Passive learning methods

PRINCIPLE

Make use of passive learning methods when you're feeling unmotivated.

Ideally, you'd like to be amazingly efficient and productive all day, every day. In practice, there are times when you won't have either the brain power or the motivation to study in the traditional sense. This is normal, don't fret. And there are still excellent ways to be productive: **passive learning methods**.

Passive learning is a way of studying that requires a lot less effort and attention than traditional methods like reading and note-taking with textbooks or lecture slides. One of the most useful methods is the use of audio. This includes listening to things like commercial lecture series, audio books, podcasts, and educational YouTube videos.

Suppose you spend a total of an hour each day commuting on the bus or subway. Instead of playing *Angry Birds* or going on Instagram, if you instead spend that time listening to your favorite commercial lecture series or medical YouTube channel, this will add up to an enormous amount of learning over time.

The beauty of passive learning methods is that it's okay even if you're not always paying full attention. Sometimes, simply being exposed to the material and catching certain phrases or principles here and there can still be fruitful. After listening to something a few times, you might be surprised how well it sticks in your mind. Sometimes, information that you *hear* can stick in your memory in ways that text cannot.

Some settings in which to consider using passive learning include while commuting, cooking or preparing food, and cleaning or doing chores.

Tip: if you're looking for subject-specific YouTube videos or series to listen to, check the respective subject's heading in the table at: **dryoumethod.com/companion_links/**

➤ 7. Building routines

Generally in life, we feel accelerations and decelerations much more than the speed we're traveling at. A billionaire, for example, having become accustomed to a lavish lifestyle, would feel highly uncomfortable for a time if he suddenly became a middle-class citizen. Meanwhile, millions of others live as middle-class citizens and are entirely comfortable with their lifestyle.

The point is, once you've become acclimated to something, it is much easier to live with. This also applies to your daily routine, and this is what you can capitalize on to steadily improve productivity in medical school.

The idea is to continuously but slowly add beneficial habits to your daily routine, such that after enough time, your day is packed to the gills with fruitful activities – all without being overly burdensome. This works so well because once something has become ingrained into your routine, you generally no longer need to actively muster up the energy to do it each time – it just becomes something you do without much thought; habit.

A prime example of this is **exercise**. For many people, it is difficult to start and maintain an exercise habit. However, if you're able to ingrain it into a *fixed* routine that you do at the exact same time each day, after some time you may well be amazed at how little conscious effort it takes. It becomes something you no longer have to psyche yourself up to do – you just do it.

The key is to add (to) those habits in small, digestible increments. In other words – going back to the momentum metaphor – increase your speed slowly so you hardly feel the acceleration. For example, if you don't exercise at all and you're struggling to implement your new plan of three 1-hour workouts per week, consider instead doing something you *know* you'll succeed at. This could be something as simple as blowing off some energy for 10-15 minutes every other day before dinner, with a quick run, skipping rope, or just jumping up and down like an idiot.

So, the take-away here is that small acts are easier to commit to routine, and once they've become routine, you can continue to slowly add more and more to them over time.

Beneficial Habits

Study-related	Outside studying
Briefly **review** that day's lecture notes the same night at roughly the same time (e.g., right before you leave school or right when you get home)	Create a simple **exercise** routine (e.g., 15 minutes of running every other day before dinner)
Listen to beneficial audio books, podcasts, or lectures while commuting	Allocating your **leisure** activities to a set time each day (e.g., one hour every day after dinner) and some to specific days (e.g., "I do not work on Friday nights after 8pm!")
Create specific daily and weekly **goals** for yourself	**Wake up** at roughly the same time each day
Summarize in your head the biggest concepts/facts you learned each day before/in bed	Be consistent with the portions of **snacks** and dessert you have each day (e.g., one chocolate bar and one small bag of chips each day)
Try a routine of **timing** work and breaks (e.g., the "pomodoro method") using a timer or app to maximize productivity and keep an honest record of your time	Eat a set amount of **fruits and vegetables** every day (e.g., one apple and one banana every day with breakfast)

> ## 8. Exercise

PRINCIPLE

Medical school is NOT a reason to abandon exercise.

One of the most absurd notions that you might come across in your peers is that you don't have time to exercise in medical school. Well, although it's probably true that mountain climbing or professional body building are not the greatest ideas, this is a myth and is counterproductive. Exercise is an essential tool to stay energetic, positive, and resilient, all of which are fundamental to doing well in medical school.

One of the greatest pitfalls surrounding fitness is the assumption that you need to devote a large amount of daily time to become and stay fit. In terms of muscle growth, for example, studies have shown that **high-intensity resistance training** can lead to muscle hypertrophy even if the exercise frequency is as little as once per week.[2]

As mentioned previously, like building any good habit, the best strategy for maintaining fitness is to incorporate exercise into a **fixed daily routine**. Exercising at the same time each day (e.g., before you eat dinner) makes it, with time, a completely normal part of your day as opposed to a chore you have to muster up the energy to perform. Whereas, if you approach an exercise schedule more openly, you will likely find it takes significantly more time and effort to decide when to do it and to motivate yourself to do it.

Additionally, to make exercise not only easier but genuinely enjoyable to maintain long term, have FUN with it. Exercise is **not** a narrow box restricted to treadmills, pushups, squats, and the like, as some imagine it. The beauty of exercise is that it's literally anything you like! So, explore different activities and see what you find most fun.

In addition to personal resistance exercises, consider things like:

- Sports (individually or as a team)
- Running or biking (consider trails or exploring new areas around you)
- Swimming
- Martial arts
- Wall climbing
- Parkour

Even if you're particularly busy on a certain day, consider simply blowing off some energy in your yard or house for 15 minutes with some high intensity movements. The important thing is to get your heart rate up, optimally above 70% of your maximum heart rate (maximum heart rate = 220 – age in years).

Remember: there are only so many hours a day you can maintain a high level of concentration

---

[2] Grgic, J., Schoenfeld, B.J., Davies, T.B. et al. (2018). Effect of Resistance Training Frequency on Gains in Muscular Strength: A Systematic Review and Meta-Analysis. Sports Med 48, 1207-1220.

crouched in a chair staring at your book or computer screen. You need to change settings and reset, and if done correctly, exercise doesn't detract from your studying, it enhances it.

Note: if you find heavy weighted exercises (e.g., heavy squats) are leaving you too fatigued to study effectively afterwards, consider decreasing the duration of the workout (e.g., number of sets) or not pushing to absolute failure.

Time-efficient strength and muscle hypertrophy training

If your specific goal is to increase strength or muscle hypertrophy, a 2021 review study by Iversen et al.[3] found a few key points for achieving optimum time-efficiency:

1. **Weekly volume** (amount of work done) is more important than training frequency. Aim for a minimum of 4 weekly sets per muscle group you're trying to work.
2. Focus primarily on **bilateral, multi-joint exercises**. It was concluded that all major muscle groups can be targeted with as few as three exercises - aim to include at least one of each:
   - Leg pressing exercise (e.g., squats)
   - Upper body pulling exercise (e.g., pullups, seated rows)
   - Upper body pushing exercise (e.g., bench press)
3. If aiming for muscle hypertrophy rather than strength, doing **supersets and drop sets** cuts training time roughly in half.
   - Superset: doing two or more exercises consecutively without rest
   - Drop set: doing a set, then reducing the load and immediately doing another set
4. Avoid extensive warmups. **Limit warmups** to a few repetitions with light loads before each exercise.
5. **Skip stretching** (unless your goal is to increase flexibility). Stretching is not necessary for strength training.

> **9. Sleep**

PRINCIPLE

Give sleep the serious attention it deserves! But if you can't sleep some nights, don't worry, you'll be okay.

There are two extremes: not giving your sleep the attention it deserves and being unrealistic by expecting perfect sleep every single night.

Overall healthy sleep habits are genuinely important in medical school for a number of reasons,

---

[3] Iversen, V.M., Norum, M., Schoenfeld, B.J. et al. (2021). No Time to Lift? Designing Time-Efficient Training Programs for Strength and Hypertrophy: A Narrative Review. Sports Med 51, 2079–2095.

including its effects on concentration, motivation, and mental health. As such, you should make a conscious effort to strive for overall adequate sleep throughout the week. On a night-to-night basis, however, some nights you might not get great sleep, and it's important to understand that that's common, okay and should not cause you to panic.

Poor sleep on a particular night might happen for various reasons, including intentionally staying up to study, stress before an exam, or simply feeling pressured to fall asleep. In any case, understand that you can generally still perform just fine on an exam with a poor night's sleep, especially if you're feeling nervous about it – that sympathetic nervous stimulation keeps you sharp during the exam! You can make up for the lost sleep later.

If you find yourself regularly experiencing stress-induced sleeplessness on nights before exams, mentally prepare yourself in advance. Recognize that it's possible you might not sleep well the night before your exam, but that it's *OKAY* and it's probably not going to significantly affect the exam's outcome. Stress sleeplessness is common amongst medical students, and even if you don't manage to change it, you *will* learn to work with it effectively and succeed regardless. Sometimes, this acceptance in itself can significantly reduce stress and improve sleep.

However, *chronically* inadequate sleep needs to be taken seriously with steps to avoid or correct it.

Evidence-based techniques to improve sleep

Four evidence-based techniques you can use to improve your overall sleep quality and/or latency:

1. Improve sleep hygiene
2. Progressive muscle relaxation (PMR)
3. Increase daytime light exposure
4. Exercise

Improve sleep hygiene

Suppose you eat dinner while watching a certain TV show every night. You might find that eventually, simply watching that show makes you hungry, even if it's not dinner time. This is called **classical conditioning**.

Apply classical conditioning to your sleep by **associating your bed with sleep and sleepiness and dissociating it from wakeful activities.**

This means reserving your bed exclusively for sleep and doing your studying and leisure activities elsewhere. Try as much as possible to only use your bed when you're actually feeling drowsy. If you can't sleep and you find yourself tossing and turning in bed for an extended time, get out of bed and return only when you're genuinely sleepy. Additionally, associate "lights on" with wakefulness and "lights off" with sleep by only turning off your lights when you're ready to get into bed.

Similarly, if you find yourself getting sleepy studying at your desk, either get up and try to shake it off or consider just going to bed. This helps maintain a strong association between your workspace and productivity.

Progressive muscle relaxation (PMR)

PMR is an evidence-based technique with a strong record of improving sleep latency (i.e., how long it takes you to fall asleep), and is even used to clinically treat insomnia. It involves three simple steps that you can do in bed:

1. While *inhaling*, contract one muscle group in your face (e.g., your forehead) for 5-10 seconds; then *exhale* and suddenly release the tension in that muscle.
2. As you release the tension, focus on the changes you feel in that muscle group as you relax it. Using imagery can be helpful, like imagining the stress flowing out of the muscles as you relax.
3. Perform the same technique for the rest of your body, from top to bottom (e.g., jaw, neck, shoulders, etc.)

Increase daytime light exposure

Studies have found that prolonged exposure to bright light during the day (e.g., natural daylight) improves both sleep quality and duration and shifts the timing of sleep to earlier hours.[4,5] In fact, it may even help offset the negative effects of prolonged screen time right before bed. It also exerts a positive influence on mood and can be beneficial as a supplement in the treatment of clinical depression.[6,7]

Bright light therapy is most effective when used on a daily basis for at least 30-60 minutes. Therefore, consider opening your curtains during the day or studying somewhere that's brightly lit.

Interestingly, a 2012 study found that even an hour of *artificial* daytime light can improve sleep patterns.[4]

Exercise

Exercise has a well-established strong association with better sleep, to the extent that its effects might be comparable to that of sleeping pills.[8,9] Specifically, aerobic exercise improves sleep

---

[4] Roenneberg T, Wirz-Justice A, Merrow M. (2003). Life between clocks: daily temporal patterns of human Chronotypes. J Biol Rhythms. 18:80–90.

[5] Corbett RW, Middleton B, Arendt J. (2012). An hour of bright white light in the early morning improves performance and advances sleep and circadian phase during the Antarctic winter. Neurosci Lett.13;525(2):146-51.

[6] Blume, C., Garbazza, C., & Spitschan, M. (2019). Effects of light on human circadian rhythms, sleep and mood. Somnologie : Schlafforschung und Schlafmedizin = Somnology : sleep research and sleep medicine, 23(3), 147–156.

[7] Martiny K. (2004). Adjunctive bright light in non-seasonal major depression. Acta Psychiatr Scand Suppl. (425):7-28.

[8] Kredlow, M. A., Capozzoli, M. C., Hearon, B. A., Calkins, A. W., & Otto, M. W. (2015). The effects of physical activity on sleep: a meta-analytic review. Journal of behavioral medicine, 38(3), 427–449.

[9] John Hopkins Medicine. (n.d.). Exercising for Better Sleep. Retrieved from https://www.hopkinsmedicine.org/health/wellness-and-prevention/exercising-for-better-sleep

latency and efficiency (the amount of time spent actually asleep while in bed).

- *Bout duration:* The research seems to show a benefit for exercise bouts of **at least 30 minutes**.
- *Intensity:* Moderate intensity (65-70% of your maximal heart rate) or above is recommended.
- *Timeline for sleep improvement:* In some, improvement in sleep is seen the very same night, while in others it may take a few days or weeks.

➤ 10. Research

Experience in research is an important quality many residency programs look for in an applicant. Many programs want residents that are not only good at patient care, but that are capable of advancing research in their field. For this reason, research experience during medical school can make you a stronger residency candidate, especially if you're hoping to apply to a competitive specialty. Your clinical years provide excellent opportunities to do so, as you tend to have more time and freedom than your basic science years.

The question though is how much, if any, time you can commit to research during your basic sciences specifically. This depends on three things:

1. How well you're **keeping up with your studies**.

    Passing and excelling in your studies is your top academic priority during your basic science years – full stop. If you're doing a reasonable job with this, you can consider research. If not, you should focus on your studies until you're in a more favorable academic position.

2. How much **competition** you'll be facing in your residency of choice.

    The more competition you'll be facing, the more advantageous it will be to get involved in research early. Specifically, there are two major factors to consider:

    a) The **specialty** you want to pursue.

    Generally, competitive specialties tend to value research more than less competitive ones. Residency programs also look for an applicant's commitment to their specialty, so doing research in that specialty is a nice way to distinguish yourself and demonstrate your commitment.

Specialty Competitiveness

Specialties with low competition (↑ supply:demand)	Specialties with high competition (↓ supply:demand)
Family medicine	Surgical specialties in general
Internal medicine	Dermatology
Pediatrics	Ophthalmology
Psychiatry	Interventional radiology
Pathology	Emergency medicine

b) Whether you're an **IMG or a native** applicant: *IMGs face greater competition.*

3. Your **genuine interest** in research

If you're genuinely passionate about doing research and wouldn't mind doing it in your free time, this is certainly an advantage and can make juggling your different responsibilities easier. If you would hate it, don't do it. There's no need to add additional stress to your already challenging basic science years. Remember: you'll likely have more free time in your clinical years and many opportunities to engage in research.

If you're pressed for time but still want to get experience in research, a smart option might be to seek out an opportunity that has a low burden of work (e.g. one that only requires you to invest a few hours per week). This is especially valuable if you're mainly pursuing research to increase your chances of matching into a competitive residency program, rather than as a genuine interest. Selection committees will look at your CV and see that your research activity spans the course of several years, and may be very impressed by this. Finding such opportunities can sometimes be tricky though, so you may have to do some exploring and emailing.

Obtaining a research position

Often the best way to obtain a research position is to simply speak to your professors, either in-person or by email, and ask them if they have any research opportunities available.

An effective strategy to increase your chances of landing a position is to write to multiple professors with a concise, well-worded and genuine email outlining who you are and why you're looking for a research position. Then, simply copy-and-paste the email to different professors, remembering to avoid dreaded copy-paste errors and **change the names!** For example:

Dear Dr./Professor _____,

I hope this finds you well.

My name is _____ and I'm a 1ˢᵗ year medical student who is really enthusiastic about getting involved in research in _____ [specialty/topic]. I know you're leading research in _____ [topic] and I wanted to kindly ask if there might be any opportunities for me to assist you in this work. I would be thrilled at the opportunity to work with you on _____!

I have prior research experience, including _____.

I would be happy to help in any capacity and have provided professional and academic references below, if needed. Thank you very much for your consideration, and I eagerly look forward to your reply.

Sincerely,

_____

Even if a particular professor doesn't have a position available, they may be able to redirect you, or even recommend you, to a professor in need of students.

Medical schools and hospitals usually have a list of faculty members and their contact information online, so search your school's (or nearby hospital's) website to see if you can find it. You might also consider reaching out to faculty at other nearby schools or research institutes.

In addition to emailing and speaking to professors, your school might have research job postings online, so do a bit of poking around to see if you can find any openings.

➤ 11. Financials

Medical school is demanding, and it is an enormous advantage if you can avoid the need to earn money. However, not everyone is so fortunate!

In such cases, a useful idea is to consider possible ways of making money that are closely related to your studies. This way, you can earn money and benefit your studies at the same time. There are a few ways of doing this, including those that pay out relatively fast and those that can generate income in the long-term.

Fast Income

The old saying, "By teaching, we learn", is quite true. By having to teach something, you're forced to really understand and remember a concept to the point that you can neatly synthesize it and explain it verbally. In doing so, your understanding of the concept becomes significantly deeper, and your memory of it becomes more fixed. This is why, if the opportunities are available, teaching or sharing your knowledge can be one of the most rewarding ways of earning money in medical school. There are a few different ways to do this, including tutoring, creating resources for different clients and research work.

Tutoring

Tutoring students in subjects you've completed can be done either by working for a tutoring company or by advertising and working independently.

- Tutoring company: Working for a tutoring company is generally easier and the income is more consistent, making it a convenient, low-stress option for medical school. Some schools have their own tutoring service that you can work for, which would be ideal.
- Independent: If you're not able to find a job with a tutoring company, you can work independently by advertising on Facebook groups (consider both your school's groups and broader groups), Craigslist, and word of mouth.

Creating educational resources

There are two types of educational resources you can create: **resources for your school** and **resources for the general market**.

Whatever you choose to sell, your focus should be on making it as high-quality as possible, rather than simply putting together something to sell. Earnings tend to go up exponentially – not linearly – with the quality of a product.

Therefore, go the extra mile and put in the time to continuously improve your product and make it as amazing as you can. Pay significant attention to details and visual appearance. Put yourself in the customer's shoes and think about what will make their experience with the product as wholesome and enjoyable as possible. It is a saying in business development that your product should address real daily problems that your customer has. As a fellow medical student, you know intimately what many of those problems are!

This level of care requires greater initial time investment, but your customers will notice and appreciate it, which will go on to pay you dividends in the near future. They'll also be excited to buy more of your products and may very well tell their friends about it. Remember: the best advertising for your product is outstanding quality.

Creating resources for your school

Resources most valuable to students at your school are those that provide them with things no mainstream resource can. In other words, rather than trying to sell them a guide to anatomy or physiology (which they can likely find a superior version of on the market), much more valuable to them would be, for example, a guide to excelling in Professor Hippityhoppity's courses, or a summary of commonly tested concepts for specific tests.

Some options include:

1. **Exam questions for each course**: One way to achieve this would be to write down every

question you remember immediately after exiting an exam, look into the correct answers, and compile them into a neat, professional-looking document. In addition to being valuable products, these serve as excellent learning opportunities for you.

2. **Guide for each course**: You'd be surprised how many students may be interested in a detailed guide for their specific course at your school. Consider including things like commonly tested areas, tips for excelling, professors' tendencies and favorite questions, and general resources to use. Consider adding in your course notes or annotated slides, if they are of good quality.

3. **Overall guide to excelling at your medical school**: There's a broad range of things to include in this. Use your creativity and think back to what would have been really helpful for you when *you* first started.

How much you charge can be highly variable and depends on a lot of factors, including what the product is, its quality, the time investment it required, and its demand. A good starting point, though, is to think about how much *you* would pay for a product similar to yours and to ask friends and family for their input.

Marketing is usually best accomplished through a combination of word-of-mouth and posting in student group chats and social media pages (e.g., Facebook). It's also beneficial, especially when you're first starting out, to give a few copies of your product out to select students for free. This helps build your credibility and sparks interest in your products. Remember to put yourself in the shoes of the customer: you're probably not going to spend money on something that you're not sure is going to help you or be worth the money.

Creating resources for the general market

Creating resources that you can sell on the general market to all medical students can be challenging because, depending on what you're creating, you may be competing with large competitors and high-quality products. The standard is therefore much higher. But the potential payoff can also be a lot higher.

Creating very generalized resources, such as a standardized exam prep book like *First Aid*, will likely be far too time-consuming for you as a medical student. Instead, use your creativity to find a niche – something specific enough that it doesn't take ages to compile, and that big-name companies and resources haven't (yet) done. For example, if you just completed your embryology course, an easy useful resource might be a compilation of the best embryology mnemonics.

Creating Resources for Your School Versus the General Market

	Resources for your school	Resources for the general market
Pros	Far less competition	Very large market
	Creating a product of genuine value is much easier	Resources more timeless*
	Marketing is much easier	Less concern of person-to-person piracy**
Cons	Small market	Greater competition
	Resources less timeless*	Standards for quality are much higher
	Higher concern of person-to-person piracy**	Effective marketing necessary

*Your school's professors, tests, content of courses, etc. can change from year to year. **Unprotected electronic resources (e.g., PDFs, PowerPoints) may be spread easily without your permission. When your market is all medical students in the world, this is much less of a concern as the few copies that might be shared are unlikely to make much of a dent in your enormous market. Furthermore, publishing options like Kindle Direct Publishing (KDP) offer good protection for electronic resources. When your market is just the students at your school, though, you will need to be more protective with your property. Remember to encrypt and password protect the file and advise your customers not to share it. Consider adding a copyright page at the start discouraging sharing of the file. Alternatively, you can consider printing the resource and selling hard copies.

Research assistant

Research experience is looked upon very favorably by most residency programs, which makes a research job a great option to make money, build your résumé, and develop valuable knowledge and skills all at the same time. Research jobs also tend to be relatively flexible in terms of hours and timing, which makes them convenient jobs for medical students. If you do pursue one, try to find a position in the specialty that you're considering practicing in. Even better is to find a specific area of research that genuinely interests you, as this will make the work even more pleasant and beneficial.

See *10. Reasearch* (page 21) for strategies in obtaining a research position.

Other Options

If the above options aren't suitable, you might consider the following jobs that tend to be convenient for medical students given the flexibility in hours and timing they offer:

1. **Non-medical tutoring**: As a medical student, you're in a good position to tutor pre-medical students for their courses or for the MCAT. As with tutoring medical school subjects, you can work for a company or independently. Big companies to consider applying to include *Kaplan*, *Varsity Tutors*, *MedSchoolCoach*, and *The Princeton Review*.
2. **Uber/Lyft**: Working for *Uber* or *Lyft* is a good option for two reasons. Firstly, it allows you to work essentially any time you wanted with no commitments, and, secondly, it can allow you time to listen to medical lectures while working (when driving non-talkative customers!).
3. **Research study participation:** While not a stable source of income, a nice bonus when available is being a participant in research studies. Researchers at universities and hospitals are regularly looking for lay participants for their studies, which can often be simple things like testing the usability of home medical devices or following a series of

instructions. Compensation is often fairly generous – typically between USD $50 and $150 per hour. To find studies, try to find out if your school and any nearby hospitals have webpages for postings, or contact research departments to ask about opportunities.

4. **Phlebotomist:** Working as a phlebotomist doesn't require any degrees or extensive training – just a certificate that typically requires around 100 to 150 hours of training. The work tends to be more flexible than many healthcare jobs and pay is around USD $15–20 an hour.

5. **Book editing**: Obtaining steady work as a book editor usually requires previous experience or a qualification. It is often another flexible type of job that allows you to work approximately when you want. You can build a profile on websites like Reedsy, Upwork or Freelancer, and accept work offers only when you want to. If you're able to get any projects editing medical books, this can also be a useful experience to highlight in your residency applications. Some medical publishers also recruit students to give feedback on material at different stages, so it can be worth reaching out to them.

Long-term income

If you don't need money right away but still want to work on setting yourself up financially for the near future (e.g., 1-3 years), the following are approaches to consider for establishing a source of **passive income**. As before, though, consider how much time this might take away from your studies. If it's a hobby that you'd like to develop in your free time, it can work. However, be cautious if it digs significantly into your study time or is in an area outside of your interest.

Creating a studygram or medical Instagram page

Creating a studygram or medical page on *Instagram* is a really simple (and fun) way of building a social media following of pre-medical and medical students that can give you a platform to run paid sponsorships from brands, as well as pursue your own entrepreneurial endeavors if you wish. Studygrams are simply pages in which the person posts visually appealing pictures of their neat little workspace, often with a caption that tells a story, shares tips, or asks engaging questions.

The idea is that as your following grows, influencers and companies reach out to you for paid promotions to advertise their product or brand. Growing your following can take some time though, and you'll likely need around 10,000 followers before you start to get a significant number of offers. Additionally, the more followers you have, the higher the pay per post. Rates vary, but one commonly cited rule is to charge USD $100 per post for every 10,000 followers you have.

The time course and income can vary significantly, but as a rough estimate: supposing you post one high-quality post every two days, a decent target for getting 10,000 followers may be 1.5 years. More effort and posts can accelerate this process.

Remember to not sell yourself out for followers though. Focus on making genuinely wholesome, high-quality posts with substance rather than simply trying to draw attention. This will pay off significantly more in the long run, as it creates an audience that is sincerely willing to support you and your work – financially or otherwise. Most importantly though, it will genuinely be better for you as a person in respect to honor and integrity.

Designing an online video course

Online video courses tend to pay quite generously, especially when they pertain to subjects that a lot of people are willing to invest money into. This can be anything, but the most glaring examples for you as a medical student are the medical school admission process, the MCAT (or UCAT for UK students), and possibly early medical school subjects, if you've attained a strong grasp of them.

If you're considering making online courses about the medical school journey, take time to think deeply about *what you wish you knew* earlier in your personal journey or what things you feel helped you immensely. Then, think about simple but unique ways of presenting that information. Continuously put yourself in the viewer's shoes and think about how you'd like the information presented if you were them.

Again, whatever you choose to teach, keep your focus on making your course as amazing as possible rather than simply putting together something just to try and sell. Also be aware that the technical and presentation skills required to make quality videos have a significant learning curve, and it takes time to do things right even once you know how. However, they are both useful skills for any medic to develop, especially presentation skills!

A course can be hosted on an online platform like Skillshare, or self-host using platforms like Teachable, Thinkific, or your own website. The difference is that in using a platform like Skillshare, you don't actually have to sell your course – people pay for a Skillshare subscription, and then Skillshare simply pays you for each minute of your course that is watched (typically between USD $0.05 and $0.10 per minute). Hosting on a platform like Skillshare is generally better if you don't already have a decent following, as the platform itself helps brings the attention of its subscribers to your course.

SECTION 3

Motivation and Mental Health

Perhaps one day, in the not-too-distant future, you'll be looking back at your tough times in medical school with a big smile on your face, proud of how far you've come and who you've become. You can't make that moment come any faster, but what you can do in the present is to improve your coping skills and use strategies to reduce stress to a minimum.

In addition to sharing some of these strategies, this section also illuminates some realities about the medical journey that will hopefully reassure you and spark optimism.

> ### ➤ 1. Things to look forward to

Clinical years are better

You didn't enroll in medical school because you love reading lecture slides and writing exams – you enrolled because you want to be a doctor and practice medicine. *Of course* you are not going to enjoy many parts of your basic sciences! Do you think any doctor out there wishes they were back in their basic sciences memorizing what happens after fructose-6-phosphate is phosphorylated?

So, don't feel like you're out of place and don't belong. Not having the most enjoyable experience now *does not* at all mean that you will dislike your life in medicine, or even your future time in medical school.

In particular, clinical years are significantly more enjoyable and less stressful for the following reasons.

Practicing real, hands-on medicine

It's frustrating to constantly dream about practicing actual medicine but be stuck in classrooms learning the basics – especially for subjects that may not seem super relevant to what you want to practice as a physician. In clinical rotations however, you are on the front lines seeing real-life cases and procedures and being a part of them too!

Much more social life

Working with other human beings on a daily basis can be a real breath of fresh air compared to studying books and slides all day. You crack jokes and laugh with colleagues and patients; you meet interesting people; you have the satisfaction of treating and comforting real patients and seeing them improve in front of you; you tackle problems as a team, and more. These social aspects undoubtedly make your work more enjoyable and rewarding.

Far fewer exams

In general, clinical years tend to have far fewer exams than the basic sciences. For example, in contrast to your weekly basic science exams, each core rotation (which usually lasts 6-12 weeks) might have just one or two end-of-rotation exams. In many schools, *elective* rotations don't even have exams at all! This significantly reduces stress.

It is much harder to fail

As mentioned above, clinical rotations rely less on exams and much more on things like your preceptor's evaluation, attendance, and completion of simple homework like patient logs and notes, online cases, etc. Put simply, if you show up every day, put in a relatively decent effort while you're there, and do a wee bit of studying at home, it's generally pretty hard to fail.

More exploratory

In the basic sciences, for the most part, every student must learn the exact same information. In clinical rotations, however, although there are standard principles and facts you must learn in each core specialty, there's also a lot of freedom to learn about whatever interests you. For example, if you're doing your core surgery rotation and you want to learn more about trauma, you can take up the trauma patients that present to the emergency department, choose trauma surgeries to scrub into, and pick the brains of the trauma surgeons you work with. You can also do elective rotations in essentially whatever specialties you like, and in different cities or even countries if you choose!

The point is to be patient and keep your chin up, champ – you have a lot to look forward to!

The basic sciences become more enjoyable

The "building block" subjects (e.g., biochemistry, histology, etc.), which are more distanced from real-life clinical practice, are generally taught at the beginning of your basic sciences. As you progress, though, what you learn becomes closer and closer to actually diagnosing and treating a patient, which is very exciting. You start to delve deeper into important diseases, medications and treatments, imaging studies, and other captivating stuff. So, if you find yourself frustrated with the content of your studies early on, keep in mind that you have a lot to look forward to – even within the basic sciences.

New experiences are most difficult in the beginning

In life in general, major changes are most difficult to cope with in the beginning. Think back to any big, stressful changes in your life, and try to remember how you felt in the beginning compared to how you feel about it now. The reality is, big changes are scary, especially when you can't yet visualize how you'll adjust to them or cope. Almost invariably, though, those early feelings of fear or sadness dissipate with time.

One of the biggest pitfalls you can therefore make in such times is to assume that the level of difficulty and stress you face at the start of your journey is going to be your new normal, leading to a bleak future. Regardless of how difficult or stressful the early days of your medical journey may seem, understand that (1) it's normal to feel scared or sad – you're not alone in feeling that way, and (2) your experience will become more comfortable with time. So don't assume your future is gloomy and depressing!

The brunt of the difficulty will pass, so be patient and don't be saddened or feel hopeless. As much as your mind is telling you you're screwed and that everything will be miserable, trust that these thoughts and emotions are part of the normal psychological process in any major, and therefore stressful, change. These hardships also build character and help carve you into a stronger person in ways you otherwise would not be able to, so recognize that there's value in them.

Additionally, if you're encountering academic difficulties early on and you aren't happy with your results, avoid the mental mistake of assuming that's how the rest of your medical education will go. Many students who struggle early on go on to do very well as they progress through their basic sciences. The early days of medical school are a lot about adjusting rather than smarts, so don't feel like you "don't have what it takes" if you find yourself struggling.

You feel better as you become more competent

You're almost guaranteed to feel lost a great deal of the time while learning medicine. It's not just you – everyone feels that way. You're essentially tasked with solving an enormous jigsaw puzzle, one tiny piece at a time.

So, rest assured: you're not lost because you're stupid or incompetent - you're lost because *everybody* is lost. Your job is simply to become a little less lost with time. This is a *long* process, so don't be discouraged by how you keep forgetting facts or how you can't seem to grasp certain concepts. Those facts and concepts come up again and again, each time strengthening your memory and allowing you to understand them in a different light. With time, your understanding of how to actually diagnose and treat patients starts to really come together, just like how a jigsaw puzzle starts to make sense and become whole. And when it does, *oof*, can it start to feel pretty sweet…

Therefore, don't be disheartened by how little you feel you know right now. As your grasp of medicine slowly starts to improve, your journey begins to feel more and more satisfying. Before you know it, you'll start answering some of your friends' and family's medical complaints and questions and start recognizing and understanding different diseases you encounter in real life. And as you do, you can't help but feel proud of how far you've come. That "Hey, I'm kind of starting to feel a bit like a real doctor" feeling that you'll get is truly indescribable.

> **2. Dealing with early disadvantage**

PRINCIPLE

The playing field becomes more level with time.

The earlier semesters of medical school can be particularly intimidating because some students may appear to have enormous advantages based on their prior studies and experiences.

You may encounter former nurses who are miles ahead of you in clinical skills, and who are already familiar with all the major medications and the "culture of healthcare". There might be kinesiology or physiotherapy graduates for whom anatomy is a breeze, or former pharmacy students who show off their knowledge in pharmacology. To a new student without such advantages, starting completely fresh, seeing these students succeed with ease early on can be very intimidating and disheartening.

However, a reality of medical school that should give you comfort is that the playing field generally becomes more level with time. Some students' prior experiences may give them advantages with certain introductory subjects, but undoubtedly your studies will progress to content that is relatively new for *everybody*. Additionally, the speed at which studies progress in medical school and the overall amount and diversity of content makes any advantages from past studies very short lived. They tend to eventually be overshadowed by the colossal scope of medicine!

In fact, sometimes those who appear to be passing with flying colors early on go on to struggle a lot when they encounter subjects they don't have prior experience with. Therefore, if you're one of those students starting off with few or no advantages, be patient early on and know that your peers' advantages will likely start to fade in a very short time.

➤ 3. Dealing with failure

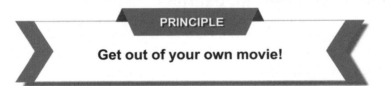

PRINCIPLE

Get out of your own movie!

If you're feeling devastated after failing a test or even an entire course, try this exercise: take a little stroll around the streets and shops in your area and observe the people you see along your way. Take a mental note of what they're doing, where they're going, how they're acting, etc.

You'll probably see a lot of things – perhaps an old lady carrying her groceries home, or a man watering his lawn and drinking lemonade, or a woman walking her dog and picking up its poop, or a young boy waiting for the bus after school. Eventually, you'll come to one very important realization: everything's fine.

Everything is fine around you and life is going on as normal. It's only your mind that's envisioning disaster, panic, and gloom. In essence, you've created a scary "movie" of your situation inside your head that you're playing over and over again – a movie that doesn't match the reality of your situation. You're imagining your dreams of practicing medicine coming crashing down, or being an incapable medical student, or being completely miserable re-taking a course.

It's this movie that's contributing to the bulk of your stress. You need to get out of that movie and turn your attention to the present *reality* around you. That is, you're going to shower and eat dinner tonight; you'll probably go on your phone or computer and browse the internet a bit; you're going to sleep in your bed, and maybe have a nice little poop in the morning when you wake up. You're okay and so is life around you.

The reality is that you likely made some simple mistakes. You zigged when you should have zagged and you ended up with an undesirable grade. *So what?* You're not the only one that has ever failed a test or course. Most of us do at some point. You need to take this test or course for what it really is: a very small stepping stone in your grand journey of practicing medicine.

Failing absolutely does *NOT* mean you've ruined your chances at a competitive residency program, so take a breath and relax. First of all, basic science grades don't mean much to most residency programs, so if you've failed a test, just take a chill pill and focus on passing the course. If you've failed a course, understand that there have been many students who have failed courses that have matched to excellent residency programs – some having even tanked entire semesters!

What residency programs really care about is your explanation of the lessons you learned from your failure and how you bounced back.

> ➤ 4. Managing anxiety before/during exams

Anxiety just before, and during, exams

Regardless of how experienced you become with exams, you will likely always experience some level of stress and anxiety before and during them. It's important to realize that this is (1) okay, (2) entirely normal and, (3) with the right attitude, beneficial.

Anxiety can either paralyze you or serve as your turbo engine to take your performance to the next level. The difference between these two outcomes is your interpretation of the anxiety.

As unpleasant as the anxiety might feel, understand that it is in fact your *friend*. Anxiety is the normal physiologic response to an important challenge lying ahead of you, and it's what keeps you sharp throughout that challenge. Instead of fighting it and trying to convince yourself that there's no need to be anxious, try to embrace it; lean into it. It's on your side, stupid – allow it to help you.

This realization on its own is often enough to make things significantly more pleasant and beneficial. However, understand that reframing your anxiety is a *skill* and takes time to polish, so continue to work on it and don't be disheartened if it takes you some time to see results.

Anxiety days or weeks before your exam

Mild anxiety the day before an exam – or even a few days before a big exam – that slowly increases as the test approaches is normal and can help motivate hard work. Excessive or persistent anxiety, though, can be debilitating and very unpleasant. If you find you consistently have persistent or excessive anxiety, see *Managing chronic anxiety and stress,* below.

> ## 5. Managing chronic anxiety and stress

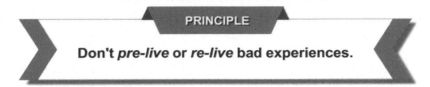

PRINCIPLE

Don't *pre-live* or *re-live* bad experiences.

Bad things *can* happen in some students' medical journeys once in a blue moon. Dropping out, failing a standardized exam, encountering difficulty matching into your specialty and other scenarios are not impossible. How can you reconcile with that fact and not allow it to terrify and paralyze you? The answer involves two steps:

1. Only live through a bad experience **ONCE**.
2. Turn your attention to the **present**.

Only live through a bad experience ONCE

Consider, for example, the fear of driving. It's important to take all the necessary steps in your power to avoid an accident, like driving at a moderate speed, avoiding distractions, etc. Nonetheless, despite all precautions, it's impossible to completely negate the risk. If it *were* to happen though, you only want to live through it **once**.

What you *do not* want to do is **pre-live** such an accident, such that every time you get into a car or think about driving you become terrified by thoughts of an accident that hasn't even happened. You also don't want to **re-live** a past accident, experiencing its distress over and over again in your mind.

By pre-living or re-living it, you essentially live through thousands of car accidents in your life and experience its agony countless times over. On the other hand, even *if* it did ever happen, in reality, it would only be once. The same can be said for bad events along your medical journey.

How do you avoid pre-living or re-living such events?

Turn your attention to the present

Focusing on the present *does not* mean forgetting about planning diligently for the future and working very hard towards it. It also doesn't mean to disregard learning from your past mistakes. Rather, it means to avoid *negative thoughts* about the future or past by focusing on the immediate task at hand, which will usually be something mundane and achievable.

For example, suppose you have a huge exam coming up. Rather than constantly thinking about how pressed for time you'll be on the exam or wondering how you'll be able to sleep with all that stress the night before, focus on *right now*. Perhaps right now you simply have to eat lunch;

after that, maybe you have to go to a lecture, say hi to your friends, and learn about the muscles of the hand from your favorite professor; after that, you might take a nap, etc.

This same principle can be applied to an exam day as well. For example, rather than envisioning the exam the entire day, focus again on your immediate task at hand: simply eating breakfast; then walking to the test center; then preparing your ID for the examiners; then tackling the single question in front of you; then the next, etc. One step at a time.

The point is: plan diligently for the future, but after you've done so, focus on the immediate task in front of you. This is a *skill,* and it takes practice, so keep working at it.

> **6. Dealing with self-doubt**

At some point along this journey, you might have asked yourself, "Do I have what it takes?" If you've doubted whether you do, don't panic.

Regardless of what others say aloud and the game faces they put on, most medical students experience self-doubt. One study at Johns Hopkins University School of Medicine of students, whom many would think of as exceptionally bright and capable, found that 71% reported self-doubt, with 69% of these students classing their doubt as moderate or severe. [10] Over half of students doubted their ability to succeed in the academic environment of medical school.

The point is: it's not just you.

Intellectual self-doubt

If your question is "Do I have what it takes *intellectually*?", the answer, if you've made it to medical school, is: it's *highly likely* that you do. The reality is that you were objectively selected to enter a medical school because you were judged intellectually qualified based on a wide range of predictive parameters. In other words, an entire team of experienced individuals, who have seen thousands of medical students over the years, have judged that you have what it takes to succeed both in medical school and at being a doctor.

You also might have heard the saying regarding the material in medical school: "it's not hard – there's just a lot of it". This is indeed true. Unlike subjects like advanced mathematics or quantum physics, most of medicine is not particularly difficult to grasp. Your success is therefore a lot more closely related to the amount of time you invest into learning and the academic strategies you use – both of which you have control over and can continually improve.

Practicing medicine as an actual doctor is a lot simpler than you might think too. Learning the information is the hard part, after which you mostly see the same things over and over again. It's like speaking a language once you've become fluent in it – it becomes second nature.

---

[10] Liu, R., Carrese, J., Colbert-Getz, J., Geller, G., & Shochet, R. (2015). "Am I cut out for this?" Understanding the experience of doubt among first-year medical students. Medical teacher, 37(12), 1083–1089.

Emotional self-doubt

If your question, on the other hand, is "do I have what it takes *emotionally*?", understand that your comfort and confidence with life in medical school is not something that you either have or don't – it's something that you can develop. In other words, even if you consider yourself an emotionally sensitive person, you can make the emotional struggle of medical school far less taxing on you by learning to make small, positive changes to different parts of your day. This way, life in medical school doesn't *need* you to fight emotionally most of the time.

To do so, think of optimizing your day in two ways: reducing stress and increasing enjoyment, often with just little techniques that can make a big difference.

Reducing stressors

For example, if you find going to class is unpleasant, study independently. If you're hating a particular subject, search for a resource that makes it slightly more palatable. If you're away from your family and you're missing them, see if you can have them on video call in the background while you study. The point is, take some time to think about what's really making you unhappy, and then think about how you might be able to decrease that a bit. It doesn't have to (and often won't) eliminate the stressor entirely, but even a slight change to a major stressor could make a world of difference.

Adding enjoyment

As with reducing stressors, adding enjoyment to your day and to your tasks doesn't have to involve big changes. Often, it's the little things that change your perception of an experience. These can be simple actions like having a nice hot or cold drink with each study session, playing comforting white noise while you study, or chatting with your friend during breaks (see *Making Studying Enjoyable* on page 10).

Use your creativity to find clever ways to reduce stressors and add enjoyment. You'd be surprised what you're able to come up with if you devote some time specifically to brainstorming solutions.

Of course, doing this doesn't eliminate emotional struggles altogether. You will almost certainly experience times that you will find very draining and emotionally challenging. But by optimizing the different pieces of your day, you can reduce how often these occur.

When you do encounter such times, remember that, as painful and drawn out as it may seem, it *will* pass. What will remain, however, are its fruits – a strengthened character, invaluable lessons to teach others, an experience that you look back at with pride, and stories to tell your grandchildren.

> **7. Keeping company while studying**

In contrast to your clinical years, your basic science years can sometimes feel isolating. As you spend large amounts of time doing individual activities like reading, completing practice questions, and the like, you can start to feel lonely. There are a few techniques that can help.

Study with friends

Studying with friends for a portion of your study time can provide an excellent source of company. The key, of course, is to do so in a way that is not significantly distracting or inefficient. An alternative is to study while a friend or family member is on video call in the background. You don't even need to speak to them – simply having them in the background while they do their thing and you do yours can give you a warm sense of company.

Study in a public area

Studying in a calming public area like a quiet coffee shop or library is a useful way of keeping company when studying with friends is inefficient or distracting. Even if you're not actively socializing with those around you, the psychological comfort of simply having people around you can be profound.

Comforting sounds

If you're studying alone, one option is to play videos or audio in the background that is comforting, e.g., white noise, nature sounds, library sounds, or ASMR. Creating dedicated study playlists on YouTube or a streaming platform can be worth the effort – just make sure it is working and not distracting you! Even simulated (good!) company can be surprisingly consoling. Playing barely audible radio (e.g., local news) in the background can also give you a pleasant feeling of being connected with the rest of the world.

> **8. Dealing with intimidation**

PRINCIPLE

Learn to see through fearmongering culture.

One thing you'll come to know early in medical school, if you haven't already, is that medical students *love* to complain. If they get through a class or semester that was difficult for them, they tend to bask in their own success by telling more junior students how "devastatingly hard" that class or semester is. For first semester students, it might be tall tales about how *brutal* the anatomy final exam is. After that, it may be chilling warnings about how *impossibly intense* neurology and pathology are, or how difficult it is to pass semester X. After that, it's complaints about the exit exam or the USMLE step 1.

What these students usually don't realize is just how harmful their words are to those they're "advising". So, I'll tell you something I wish more people told me when I was a wee lad in first year:

Take everyone's fearmongering and intimidation with a grain of salt.

The challenges throughout medical school are all *MANAGEABLE!* Of course, there are some courses and semesters that are more demanding than others, but don't let *ANYONE* shake your confidence with their cautionary tales. Realize that there's *always something* that some medical students will complain about. Get used to hearing such "warnings" and learn to simply brush them aside. If you don't, your anxiety may constantly eat away at you and make your medical school experience unnecessarily difficult. Instead, just focus on tasks at hand, and try to have fun with them!

It's also a smart strategy to find a senior mentor who's not only knowledgeable but also encouraging and supportive.

NOTES

SECTION 4

Overall Basic Science Strategies

Think of your academic success in terms of two things: (1) the **amount of time** you spend studying, and (2) the **strategies** you use.

You can increase your study time to a certain extent, but ultimately, everyone shares the same number of hours in a day. Using the right strategies, on the other hand, can significantly increase the efficiency with which you study, essentially freeing up substantial amounts of time for you in the long run; more time for study or relaxation. So consider the strategies in this section carefully and remember that many of them are skills that take time to be honed, so practice them and don't be disheartened if it takes time to grasp them.

➤ 1. School grades vs. standardized exam scores

In the basic sciences, you have to strike a balance between preparing for school exams (i.e., attending lectures and studying lecture slides) and standardized exams (e.g., completing test banks, using supplementary resources, etc.) Although most of the content between school and standardized exams overlap, not all of it does.

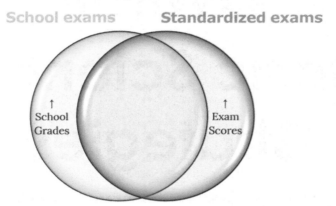

Preparation time.

The reality is that you need to pass school exams in order to pass your courses and progress to the next semester. There won't *be* any standardized exams to take if you don't get through your courses! For that reason, first thing's first: get to a position where you're reasonably confident that you'll pass your course, after which you can devote increasingly greater time to standardized exam preparation.

For example, suppose your pathology course has a total of four block exams. You may consider devoting your study time for the first two exams mostly to the content on those exams, trying to ensure you achieve high grades (i.e., making sure you know your professor's slides very well). If you do quite well on those two, you then have a decent "cushion" in the course, which can give you some time to focus on standardized exam content for your remaining two blocks. For example, suppose your third block is centered on respiratory pathology – you can devote a greater chunk of your study time to completing practice questions (e.g., Kaplan, UWorld) and a little bit less to memorizing lecture slides. If you again excel on your third exam, you may devote even more time to standardized exam content for block four.

> **2. Approach guidelines**

PRINCIPLE

**Assume your approach is flawed
(probably much more than you think).**

The importance of continuously refining your methods and approaches in the basic sciences cannot be overstated. One of the most disastrous mistakes a student can make is to cling onto a strategy that they've grown comfortable with or that worked for them in the past, despite it not *currently* producing results. Students may often realize far down the line that it wasn't exactly as spectacular as they imagined, but by then the damage has been done.

For example, some students learn about the use of mnemonics – a genuinely useful tool when used appropriately – and then start to use them for anything and everything. A lesson you will learn, however, regardless of whether you reflect on your strategies or not, is that some things are better learnt without mnemonics. Reflection significantly speeds up the learning of that lesson. You would much rather come to that conclusion early and on your own rather than wait for a failed course or semester to tell you so.

Therefore, go in with the mindset that your approach is flawed – likely more than you think – and that your job is to make it less flawed over time. You do this by regularly reflecting on the results that a particular strategy is giving you. If it's not producing the desired results, you need to either discard it or think about how you can improve it. If your textbook isn't working for you, turn to *Google* or *YouTube* videos. If attending lectures aren't proving too fruitful, study on your own. If your memorization techniques are too slow, let them go. The point is, be willing to give any strategy or resource up.

For studying strategies in particular, questions to keep in mind are:

- How fast do you learn the information with it (or: how much time investment does it require)?
- How well do you remember the information in the short and long term with it?
- Does it improve your overall understanding of the subject?
- How have your test scores been since using it?
- Does it make the process of studying any more or less pleasant?

Not all of the answers to the above questions have to be positive. However, these are some factors that should weigh into your decision to continue or discontinue a strategy.

> **3. Test-taking strategies**

Approach to reading questions

Read questions in the following order:

1. Last sentence of the question stem (usually the question itself)
2. Entire question stem
3. Answer choices

There are a couple of reasons for following this order. Firstly, knowing the question beforehand helps keep you sharp and efficient when reading the question stem because it makes your reading goal-directed. Especially for longer vignettes and after you've been through numerous questions already, your attention and reading speed start to fade. It then becomes easier to skip over important details or go over time. On the other hand, knowing the question you're trying to answer gives you something specific to search for and a reason to really care about what you're reading.

Secondly, some questions waste your time by giving you a vignette with unnecessary context. For example, they might tell you all about a confused 67-year-old patient who has this past history and is presenting with these signs and symptoms, and then ask you, "Which of the following is an expected imaging finding in Alzheimer disease?"

By reading the last sentence first, you can quickly identify questions that you don't need to read the vignette for. The time you save can add up to be significant, especially in exams in which you're pressed for time.

Reading the answer choices before the question stem carries a risk of making you biased as to what you are looking for and how you value and interpret findings. While this might not be a major issue for questions in which you're reasonably sure of the answer, it might throw off your sense of intuition for questions you are uncertain of (which is quite common!) Instead, as you read the question stem, try to first formulate an answer to the question *on your own*. If you see your answer listed as an answer choice, this increases the likelihood of it being correct.

Images

If the question has an image of a physical finding, imaging study, or pathology specimen, look at the image first for a few seconds at most, and see if you can figure out what the disease is. Often, you can figure out the answer from the image alone or at least get a good hunch. This hunch is valuable because you haven't yet been influenced by the question stem (which is sometimes meant to trick you). You can then use the image and the question stem as two independent pieces of evidence to come to a conclusion.

Note: this does NOT apply to ECGs or complicated graphs. These take longer to interpret, and if you don't know exactly what you're looking for you very well might waste a lot of time.

Timeouts

When you're panicking or just getting into a really bad flow, take a deep breath and consider taking a timeout of up to 30 seconds. Negative thinking patterns can significantly hurt both your speed and your ability to find the right answers. Therefore, breaking this pattern and clearing your head with a short timeout may well be worth a lot more than the 30 seconds it takes to do so. Use this time to:

1. **Breathe** slowly and focus on your breathing.
2. **Let go** of what has already passed.
3. **Encourage yourself** with positive thoughts.

Guessing

For questions in which you simply have no clue what the answer is, first eliminate any obviously incorrect or unlikely options, and then go with your gut feeling. If you have no gut feeling, **choose the answer choice that looks most familiar to you**. This will usually serve you better than choosing an answer that's more obscure or unfamiliar.

Another tip: if two answer choices are the opposite of each other, the correct answer tends to be one of these two.

Changing your answer

- If you're changing your answer because you re-read the question and found some new information or understood it in a new way, go with your **new answer**.
- If you're changing your answer because you're just torn between two choices, it helps if you have some evidence of how good of a second-guesser you are. You can assess this with feedback from most major question banks, as they report your correctness percentage for questions in which you changed your answer. If your second-guesses are wrong more often than not, or if you just don't have this information, it's probably best to stick with your **original answer**.

> **4. Memorization-heavy vs. understanding-heavy subjects**

PRINCIPLE

Review understanding-heavy info earlier on, and memorization-heavy info closer to the exam.

Ideally, strive for understanding over brute memorization whenever possible. However, there are undoubtedly some things that simply have to be memorized. This information tends to be easier to review but also easier to forget. On the other hand, information that relies more on understanding is not as easily forgotten but generally requires greater initial time commitment to learn. Therefore, when preparing for a test, review understanding-heavy info earlier on, and memorization-heavy info closer to the exam.

Understanding-heavy vs. memorization-heavy subjects

Subjects heavier in simple memorization	Subjects heavier in understanding
Pharmacology	Pathology
Microbiology	Physiology
Anatomy	Ethics
Biochemistry	Epidemiology / biostatistics
Nutrition	Immunology

For each subject in this book, a rating out of 5 is provided for how memorization-heavy it is at the beginning of the chapter.

➤ 5. Mnemonics

Mnemonics are any tool that aids memory, like humorous sayings that signify an acronym. They can be invaluable tools, if used *wisely*. However, they can be counter-productive if used inappropriately.

Mnemonics to avoid

Avoid long "phrase" mnemonics as much as possible. These are meant to help you remember a series of words by using the first letter of each word to come up with a whacky phrase. For example:

Branches of the external carotid artery:

Some Angry Lady Figured Out PMS =

Superior thyroid, **A**scending pharyngeal, **L**ingual, **F**acial, **O**ccipital, **P**osterior auricular, **M**axillary, **S**uperficial temporal.

Although occasionally useful, these are generally **bad mnemonics**.

There are too many layers of information, and a crack in one of these layers means the mnemonic becomes essentially useless when you need it. In other words, it requires you to perfectly remember what the phrase is, what it's supposed to represent (e.g., external carotid branches), and finally what medical word each letter is supposed to represent. It's too non-intuitive, and after some time there's a high likelihood of forgetting parts or all of it.

Instead, try your best to find any logical reasoning or meaningful connections between the items. If all else fails, simple brute repetition is usually still more effective than these phrase mnemonics.

Mnemonics to use

Play-on-words mnemonics

Spend some time thinking about the word you're trying to memorize and see if you can find another word that <u>sounds similar</u> *and* <u>relates to its meaning</u>.

> a. E.g., a **fun**dus is a **fun**nel-shaped structure

This way, whenever you see the word (e.g., *fundus*), you remember the other word (*funnel*) and hence its meaning.

"People's names" mnemonics

Many medical terms, including diseases, clinical signs, and tests, are named after actual people. These can be very frustrating because they are completely non-descriptive – the name gives you no hint as to what the actual thing is. In these cases, you have two useful options:

1. If the name sounds like an object, you can use a play-on-words mnemonic as described above.

> b. E.g., **Boer**haave syndrome is a transmural rupture of the esophagus, so think "*bore* a hole through the esophagus".

2. Picture someone you know with that name.

> c. E.g., **Wilson's** disease is a disorder in copper metabolism causing copper accumulation in your body – so picture your friend **Wilson** working in a copper mine.

Short, intuitive first-letter mnemonics + imagery

Take the first letter of each of the words you need to memorize and see if it forms a word that you can somehow relate to what you're trying to memorize. Then, visualize it.

> d. E.g., Calf muscles (superficial to deep): **G**astrocnemius, **P**lantaris, **S**oleus = **GPS** (then imagine a **GPS** tracker around your **calf**)

This differs from the "long phrase mnemonics" discouraged earlier because this mnemonic actually relates to the facts you're trying to memorize (GPS tracker around your *calf* helps you remember the *calf* muscles).

Intuitive rhyme mnemonics

Although these tend to not be the most effective mnemonics when you think of them on your own, some well-established rhyme mnemonics, especially when narrated to you by someone else, can be very memorable.

> e. E.g., Innervation of the diaphragm: *"C3-5 keeps the diaphragm alive!"*

Number mnemonics

If you have to memorize a small number and there's no reasoning to understand behind it (e.g., what chromosome number a disease is inherited on), you have two valid options: **brute repetition** or a **number mnemonic**. See what works better for YOU.

To create a number mnemonic, think of a common association with the number in question and see if you can visually relate the item to the number. For example:

> ➤ Fact to memorize: Hearing is innervated by cranial nerve 8.
> ➤ Mnemonic: Picture **hearing** the cracking sound of striking the **8-ball** in billiards.

This technique works well for lower numbers (e.g., 12 or less) but not so much with higher numbers (unless you can find a meaningful association with that number).

Common associations with numbers

Number	Common Associations
1	Winner/first-place/gold medal Picking nose
2	Peace sign Anything that occurs in pairs (pants, shoes, headphones, scissors)
3	OK-sign Three amigos
4	Glasses ("four-eyes") Four-leaf clover
5	Hand (five fingers) Five Guys (restaurant)
6	Dice Sixth sense Six Flags (theme park)
7	Seven deadly sins 7-Up (soft drink) Calendar (i.e., 7 days of the week)
8	8-ball (billiards) After Eight (chocolate)
9	Cat ("nine lives")
10	Dime "X marks the spot"
12	Dozen eggs Clock

The numbers 1, 2, and 10 are fairly easy numbers to remember without mnemonics. Therefore, see if brute memorization works better for you for remembering these.

Another useful way to remember numbers is to perform an action with that number of fingers on your hand that is related to the fact. These are often not readily do-able, but when they are, they can be extremely valuable. For some odd reason though, these stop working so well after the number 10.

Example 1: Smell is innervated by cranial nerve **1** → pick your nose with **1** finger.

Example 2: Sensation of the face is innervated by cranial nerve **5** → wipe your face with your hand (**5** fingers).

➤ 6. How to memorize something

Memorization techniques, from best to worst

Order	Technique	Example
1	Understanding the actual reasoning	Rib fractures predispose to pneumonia because patients take shallow breaths due to pain, which allows bacteria to grow undisturbed
2	Finding a logical pattern between items	The 3 branches of the celiac artery (common *hepatic*, left *gastric*, and *splenic* arteries) correspond to the 3 major organs in that vicinity (*liver, stomach, spleen*)
3a	Play-on-words mnemonic	A fundus is a funnel-shaped structure. Boerhaave syndrome (transmural esophageal rupture) → think: "bore a hole through the esophagus"
3b	High-quality visual mnemonic	Sketchy Medical
4	Short, intuitive first-letter mnemonic + imagery	Calf muscles (superficial to deep): GPS = Gastrocnemius, Plantaris, Soleus (then imagine a GPS tracker around your calf)
5a	Intuitive rhyme mnemonic	Innervation of the diaphragm: "*C3-5 keeps the diaphragm alive!*"
5b	Brute repetition alone	-
6	Long "phrase" mnemonic	External carotid artery branches: Some Angry Lady Figured Out PMS = Superior thyroid, Ascending pharyngeal, Lingual, Facial, Occipital, Posterior auricular, Maxillary, Superficial temporal

Regardless of what technique you use, **there is no way around repetition**. You must encounter the information you've learned at least once more in order to effectively anchor it into your memory.

> ➤ 7. 11 Strategic principles

Eleven Strategies for Memorization	
1. **Focus on names**	The name of something often tells you exactly what it is
2. **Think about the logic**	Understanding the reasoning behind something makes it significantly easier to remember
3. **Compartmentalize information**	Clusters of information are much easier to remember than scattered facts
4. **Look at the forest, then the trees**	First try to understand a new concept at its most basic level
5. **Principle-seeking**	Take your time to understand a new principle
6. **Visualization**	Visualize it!
7. **Spaced repetition**	Review information at increasingly spaced intervals
8. **Recall is better than recognition**	Test your recall before you look back at your notes
9. **Number things**	Number related facts when learning them
10. **"Questionify"**	As you learn, write new facts in the form of a question to test yourself later
11. **Correct your mistakes immediately after the exam**	Your memory is most receptive to correcting mistakes right after exams

1. Focus on names

 PRINCIPLE

The name of something often tells you exactly what it is.

Medicine is a lot like learning a new language. Thousands of times over, you must link a new word to a concept in your mind. What is very often overlooked in doing this is that, hiding in plain sight, the word itself often describes the concept.

Therefore, one of the most valuable principles for all of medical school is to make a conscious effort to think about the name of whatever you're learning. Surprisingly frequently, you'll find that the name tells you the exact information you're looking for. And this makes it much easier to remember.

For example, take neurodevelopmental disorders: *anencephaly, holoprosencephaly, encephalocele, spina bifida occulta, meningocele,* & *meningomyelocele.* It might seem like a headache to learn, but think carefully about their names and they'll tell you exactly what you need to know.

Neurodevelopmental disorders

Word	Etymology	Therefore
Anencephaly	*'a-'* means *'without/not'* (e.g., atypical); *'-cephaly'* means *'brain'*	**born without a forebrain**
Encephalocele	*'-cele'* means *'herniation'* (you'll soon become very familiar with this word!)	**herniation of the brain**
Holoprosencephaly	*'holo-'* means *'whole'* (no surprise there); *'pro-'* means *'forward'* (e.g., *pro*gress, *pro*geny)	**forebrain remaining whole** (normally it separates into 2 hemispheres)
Spina bifida occulta	*'bifida'* means *'splitting'* (think of how *bi-* means *two*); *'occulta'* means *'hidden'*	**a hidden splitting of the spine**
Meningocele	*'meningo-'* means *'meninges'*; *'-cele'* again means *'herniation'*	**herniation of the meninges**
Meningomyelocele	*'myelo-'* means *'spinal cord'*	**herniation of the meninges *and* spinal cord**

Not too bad, right?

Remember: it takes time to build your vocabulary. This process might initially be a bit slow, but continue to work on it and it will pay off immensely as your vocabulary starts to expand.

2. Think about the logic

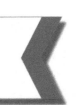

PRINCIPLE

Understanding the reasoning behind something makes it significantly easier to remember.

An idea that makes sense to you is far easier to remember than a simple fact. Memory may often fail you, but an idea with logic behind it can be worked out on the go. The actual process of reasoning the concept out also helps to solidify your memory of it. Most importantly, though, understanding the logic is immensely valuable for long-term learning as it helps you learn future related facts and concepts significantly faster. Consider the following example:

> The drug misoprostol causes **dilation of the cervix** and **contraction of the uterus**. On its own this might be easy to confuse (e.g., an answer choice on an exam might trick you with "dilation of the cervix and *relaxation* of the uterus"). But take a moment to think about it logically: it makes sense that dilation of the cervix and contraction of the uterus go hand-in-hand because this is the natural process of childbirth (**widening the opening** and **squeezing out the baby**)! This makes even more sense when you realize that misoprostol is a drug used to induce labor.

Perhaps this bit of reasoning saves you a lifetime of mix-up between misoprostol's effects. The same applies to other concepts.

Therefore, when learning new things, frequently ask yourself *"why?"*, and see if you can find a logical reason for it. It might take slightly longer to learn the new fact, but it will save you significantly more time in the long run.

Keep in mind, though, that you won't always be able to find a reasoning for everything – some things simply have to be memorized!

3. Compartmentalize information

PRINCIPLE

Groups of information are easier to remember than scattered facts.

Retaining the overwhelming amount information thrown at you in the basic sciences is very difficult if you learnt it as scattered facts. Our minds find it much easier to remember information when it's grouped into nice little compartments.

For example, the layers of the abdominal wall are (superficial to deep):

> Camper fascia, Scarpa fascia, external oblique muscle, internal oblique muscle, transversus abdominis muscle, transversalis fascia, preperitoneal fat, and parietal peritoneum.

Not so easy to memorize, right? But try categorizing it like so:

1. Two layers of **fascia** (Camper and Scarpa)
2. Three layers of **muscle** (external oblique, internal oblique, transversus abdominis)
3. **Fascia** (transversalis)
4. **Fat** (preperitoneal)
5. **Peritoneum**

A bit easier to digest and remember, isn't it?

Therefore, **search for patterns** in information where possible and use similarities to group things together. In anatomy, this might be things like a common innervation, function, location, etc. In pharmacology, it might be a common prefix or mechanism of action. In microbiology, it might be a common mode of transmission or affected organ.

4. First look at the forest, *then* the trees

PRINCIPLE

Wrap your head around what the concept is at its most basic level.

The sheer amount of detail in your basic sciences can sometimes make it difficult to come out of a lesson remembering much of anything at all. A mistake that contributes to this is focusing excessively on all the details when being introduced to a new concept, a form of information-overwhelm and loss of the ability to prioritize.

Not all information deserves equal amounts of your attention initially. Having a clear and simple image in your mind of the topic – a framework – is key to having a strong grasp of it. It also makes subsequent learning of its finer details much more efficient and enjoyable.

Therefore, when learning new concepts, begin by looking at it (the forest) from as far back as you can and simply asking yourself, "What is this thing?" Then, proceed to learn the concept in **layers of increasing detail**.

Suppose, for example, you're just starting to learn about diabetes. You can approach it like this:

1. Layer 1 (*what is diabetes even?*): Diabetes is a disease where blood glucose is chronically high, and that high glucose causes damage to all kinds of tissues.

   *That's it! Visualize that and pause to give it a moment to sink in. This is the **most important step**. When you're comfortable with that, you can add a bit more detail:*

2. Layer 2: The high blood glucose in diabetes is due to a problem with insulin – the hormone that decreases blood glucose by increasing its uptake by tissues. Type 1 diabetes is due to not making *enough* insulin, while type 2 diabetes is due to tissues becoming *insensitive* to insulin.
3. Layer 3: (even more detail, etc.)

Two tips for applying this principle in lectures are to verbalize your understanding and to prioritize the information as you digest it.

Verbalize

Consider summarizing your understanding of the concept to your professor and asking if it's correct.

Summarizing it aloud forces you to condense the concept into a simple, logical and communicable idea. It also leads to correction of any misunderstandings you have, and the process of simply vocalizing your thoughts to someone and having a discussion creates a real-life memory, which tends to stick better than thoughts floating in your mind or words on a page. Additionally, consider Googling the concept, as many of the top results you find will have crisp summaries of it (including *Wikipedia*!)

Prioritize

After each lecture, ask yourself, "*What are the big things I learned from that lecture?*"

In addition to helping reinforce the information in your memory and identifying points of confusion, plainly asking yourself what you learned helps create clarity in your mind as to what the most *valuable* information was.

5. Principle-seeking

> **PRINCIPLE**
>
> **When you stumble upon a new principle, take your sweet, delicate time.**

In your basic sciences, the bulk of the information thrown at you is simple facts, for example: *mesotheliomas* are a lung cancer associated with asbestos exposure.

Sometimes, however, you stumble upon an exciting new *principle*, for example: chronic inflammation of a tissue can lead to neoplasm. Principles are absolute medical student ***gold*** because they are the foundations that shape your entire understanding of a subject permanently, and make subsequent learning of facts significantly more intuitive.

For this reason, a critical (and unfortunately common) mistake students make, especially when going through question banks, is adhering strictly to a pace or time limit they set for themselves. Not all questions and facts you come across are equal, and some deserve a lot more attention than others. Being too strict in following a pace can therefore lead you to not spend enough time on a priceless new principle.

For example, you might spend three minutes memorizing which cancers involve the *JAK2* mutation, which you might end up forgetting anyways, and may get two exam questions on it in your lifetime. On the other hand, you might invest 10 minutes trying to understand how obstruction of any hollow organ can lead to infection, and this might change your entire understanding of medicine permanently (in addition to the *countless* exam questions you'll encounter related to this!).

In short: not all information is equal. New principles are invaluable, so be willing to give generous time to learning them when you come across them. They'll likely be immensely more timesaving in the long run than learning random facts.

6. Visualization

> **PRINCIPLE**
>
> **Visualization improves understanding and creates a more stable memory.**

A 16-year-old Albert Einstein grasped the constancy of the speed of light on his own. He credited this and many of his other revolutionary discoveries to *visualization*. He'd imagine things and visually play with them in his head - even in completely unrealistic ways - until he got a better understanding of how it worked. Similarly, he was known for his thought experiments, like imagining chasing a beam of light and considering what he would see as his own speed changed.

In a similar fashion, the basic sciences are filled with many abstract concepts, so use visualization where possible to help you understand them. Not only does this help transform a memorized fact into an understood concept, but the vivid imagery also helps create a more stable memory. As with principle-seeking, it might cost a little bit of extra time upfront, but it will save you time when reviewing. You also become more skilled at it with practice, which speeds up the process.

You don't need to try to visualize every new fact you learn, though – it would be time-inefficient to do so. Visualization is most beneficial for **physiological processes** and **anatomy**.

7. Spaced repetition

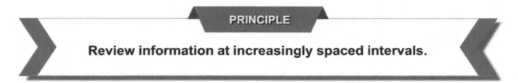

PRINCIPLE

Review information at increasingly spaced intervals.

Not all repetition is equal. A big mistake (and a huge timewaster) some students make is to review information over and over without proper spacing in between. In doing so, they may review a fact a dozen times over within two days and still likely forget it after a couple of weeks. But with strategically timed recall, three reviews might create a memory lasting months or even years.

Projected likelihood of remembering

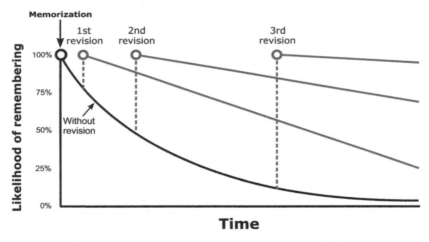

There are key points at which we tend to forget a newly learned fact. Recalling and reviewing the information at these specific points helps to consolidate it into long-term memory in the least amount of review time.

There is no consensus in the scientific literature regarding when exactly these points are, let alone how to best tailor these intervals to medical school. In reality, you need to find what works best for you and take into account factors like the time to your exam(s), level of importance of the material (i.e., low-yield information requires less repetition than high-yield information), and other time commitments and subjects.

In my experience, though, a highly effective sequence for medical school is:

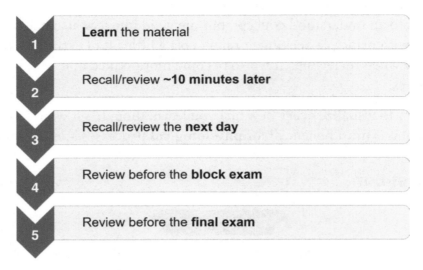

1 **Learn** the material

2 Recall/review **~10 minutes later**

3 Recall/review the **next day**

4 Review before the **block exam**

5 Review before the **final exam**

*2.5. OPTIONAL: try to briefly recall it later that night e.g. while you're in bed

A useful app to consider that helps you employ spaced repetition is *Anki* (see Page 63).

8. Recall over recognition

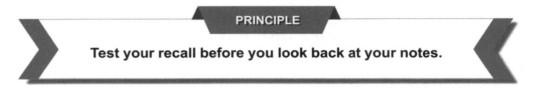

PRINCIPLE

Test your recall before you look back at your notes.

Recalling information (i.e., retrieving it from memory on your own) is superior to simply recognizing it for two main reasons:

1. Mentally reconstructing the concept or idea in your mind strengthens your memory of it significantly more than just looking at it.
2. Trying to recall something on your own identifies the gaps in your understanding.

Recognition tends to give a false sense of reassurance that you're comfortable with the information. It can also cause you to hit roadblocks when the exam presents the information from a different angle or in a different context. Recall, on the other hand, nurtures a more thorough level of understanding.

Therefore, when reviewing for an exam, avoid going straight through all of your notes and instead, look only at the headings or topics and see if you can recreate them in your mind or recall its information on your own first. *Then* look at to your notes to fill in the gaps and correct your mistakes. The very experience of realizing you made a mistake in itself also helps anchor the information into your memory.

9. Number things

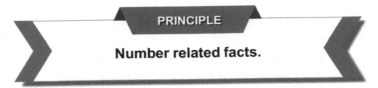

PRINCIPLE

Number related facts.

Numbering things can make them much easier both to learn and to remember for two major reasons: (1) it creates a clear mental map of exactly how many items there are in that information set, and (2) it helps creates order.

Consider points on an actual map: on their own, they're simply random points, but number them and connect the dots between them and they become a journey that you can travel along.

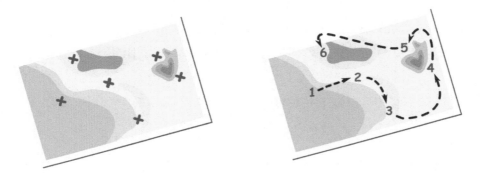

Numbering medical facts, in some ways, works similarly.

Suppose you had to memorize the branches of the facial nerve: *temporal, zygomatic, buccal, mandibular,* and *cervical.*

Now try memorizing them after numbering them. The 5 branches are:

1. Temporal
2. Zygomatic
3. Buccal
4. Mandibular
5. Cervical

Notice any difference?

10. "Questionify"

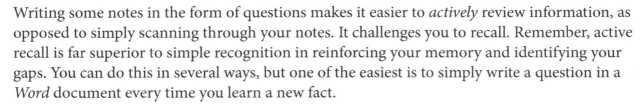

PRINCIPLE

As you learn new facts, write them in the form of questions to test yourself with later.

Writing some notes in the form of questions makes it easier to *actively* review information, as opposed to simply scanning through your notes. It challenges you to recall. Remember, active recall is far superior to simple recognition in reinforcing your memory and identifying your gaps. You can do this in several ways, but one of the easiest is to simply write a question in a *Word* document every time you learn a new fact.

For example, suppose you learn from a question in a test bank that the primary imaging test for pneumonia is X-ray. Instead of just writing a note re-stating that, you could phrase it as a question:

What's the primary imaging test for pneumonia?

> **X-ray**

When you want to review, you can scroll down the page so that only the question is visible, while the answer (i.e., the line right below it) is covered. Then, simply scroll down to see the answer. Add a star to a question each time you answer it incorrectly or feel you need more practice with it. This way, you can quickly review your weak areas before exams without wasting time on areas you're comfortable with.

Three nuances:

1. Writing questions is best for *isolated new facts*, whereas writing an organized summary or annotating your copy of *First Aid* is best for learning a *whole new concept*.

   Question-making can be used in a variety of settings, but it's perhaps most valuable when doing practice questions and adding random bits of knowledge to a foundation you *already have*. On the other hand, when learning a whole new topic or concept for the first time, it's generally more beneficial to write out an organized summary of it or annotate your *First Aid* rather than writing a bunch of questions. This is because a clean summary can organize a concept in your mind better than a set of random, scattered questions. Remember: creating order to the information you're learning is paramount.

2. Consider writing questions on a computer rather than by hand.

   If you enjoy the process of writing questions out by hand, there is nothing wrong with doing so. Enjoying your learning process

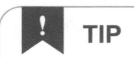

! TIP

An added perk to question-making is that once you've finished the course, you might be able to **sell these questions** and make some profit!

is invaluable to your success! However, do bear in mind time efficiency, as typing is usually significantly faster.

3. Wording matters.

    Don't be too leading with your questions – you want to provoke critical thinking. You also don't want to be overly vague, such that you don't even know what your question is specifically asking. This is something you get better at with time.

11. Correct your mistakes immediately after the exam

PRINCIPLE

After an exam, you have a golden window during which correcting your mistakes will be remembered especially well.

NOBODY likes to look at or even be in the same room as their notes immediately after an exam.

However, the benefits of spending *just a few minutes* correcting your mistakes and misunderstandings during this "golden window" period are immense. Whatever mistakes or uncertain questions you look up will stick to your memory especially well, because they will be forever linked to a real-life event that involved strong emotions and real implications. From then on, you'll think of it as "that bum fact that cost me that stupid point on that rat test".

Remember: in medical school, facts and concepts come up *again and again*, so assume you will see your mistaken questions come up in some form again in the future. So, take advantage of that golden window of heightened memorability and anchor those corrections into your mind. The next time you see that question, you can then feel joy, not frustration.

NOTES

SECTION 5

Overall
Basic Science
Resources

This section discusses general resources that are applicable to most or all basic science subjects. Subject-specific resources are reviewed in each subject's chapter in *SECTION 6: Subject Guides* (see page 69).

> ## ➤ 1. The "Big 3" resources

Three resources will likely be invaluable throughout your entire basic sciences (and in the case of the first two, throughout clinical rotations as well) – they are **YouTube**, **Google Images**, and **First Aid for the USMLE Step 1**.

YouTube

There's an immense number of content creators producing educational videos, and typically the best videos get the most views. Hence with a quick search, you can often find some of the best and easiest-to-follow explanations of medical concepts out there.

YouTube also allows you to see real-life cases of almost every disease or clinical scenario. This is invaluable in terms of solidifying your memory and understanding, as seeing something with real, vivid imagery generally leaves a much more lasting memory than words on a page.

Therefore, use YouTube to:

1. **Find high-quality explanations**
2. **See real patients with a disease**. One of the best channels for seeing real patients is Larry Mellick *(www.youtube.com/user/lmellick)*. If you see a video on the topic/disease you're looking for by him, click on it!

For each subject chapter in *SECTION 6: Subject Guides*, there are subheadings for *Useful YouTube channels* and *Useful Youtube videos and series*, respectively. These channels and videos are some of the very best on YouTube for the given subject, so consider making use of them.

If using the eBook version of this book, you can simply click on the links. If using the hardcopy version, all video and channel links are neatly listed at www.dryoumethod.com/companion_ links so that you don't have to type out the URLs manually.

Google Images

As mentioned above, seeing something is an entirely different experience from reading about it. Even with the best of resources, like your *First Aid* textbook, there is usually a limited number of quality images that authors include. With Google Images, you can find an immense number of images of almost any given thing. Some of these can be real gems.

When first learning a particular thing, try to find very **simple images** with minimal detail. This will help you understand and remember the basic idea much more than detailed images.

Searching on Google Images also tends to bring up very useful charts and comparisons between things when you search for two terms and include "versus" (e.g., *type 1 vs. type 2 diabetes*). Consider doing this whenever you'd like a clearer understanding of the differences between two or more things.

First Aid for the USMLE Step 1

First Aid for the USMLE Step 1, or *First Aid* for short, is an essential book to carry with you throughout your entire basic sciences. It is a concise book that contains the most important details of most major topics in your basic sciences. It neatly arranges each organ system into embryology, anatomy, physiology, pathology, and pharmacology subsections, and contains chapters on subjects like biochemistry, microbiology, immunology, public health sciences, etc. As such, it serves three critical purposes for your basic sciences:

1. It ensures you learn the most important information for a given topic.
2. It serves as a roadmap for each subject, ensuring that you cover the most important topics.
3. It helps you mentally organize all basic science information.

How to use First Aid effectively

1. BEFORE learning a new topic: find and read it first in *First Aid*.
   - This will usually give you a clean picture of what the topic is, as well as the most important details to focus on as you're learning it.
2. WHILE learning the new topic (e.g., during lectures): follow along in your *First Aid* and fill in any important information that's missing.
   - Over time, this will allow you to create a mental map of your entire basic sciences, making the plethora of information you've acquired all neatly organized in your mind – just as it is in your physical *First Aid* book. Make sure you don't flood each page with excessive detail though. When you open your *First Aid* book, you'd like it to be a joy to read because of how simple, memorable, and easy-to-follow it is. Pages full of your notes of non-critical facts somewhat defeats that purpose. You can store less-critical information elsewhere (e.g., a *Word* document).

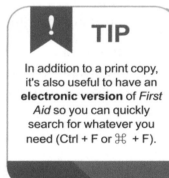

TIP

In addition to a print copy, it's also useful to have an **electronic version** of *First Aid* so you can quickly search for whatever you need (Ctrl + F or ⌘ + F).

> **2. Anki**

Another resource that many students find useful for reviewing information is **Anki**.

Anki is an app that allows you to create flashcards (or use other people's flashcards) and review them using spaced repetition. The intervals at which you review each card are based on how you rate your comfort level with it. For example, if you answered a card wrong, you can choose "Again" and it will be shown to you again in a short time (e.g., 1 minute); or, you can rate it

"Good" and it will be shown to you the next day, for example; or, you can rate it "Easy" and it will be shown to you at an even later interval. You can adjust these intervals yourself.

Overall, Anki can be a very useful tool, but it is a matter of preference and is not essential. The process of card-making can also be time-consuming. What might be more advantageous is either (a) using pre-made decks (there are some excellent ones out there), or (b) simply writing out your questions in a *Word* document and writing the answers below them (cover up the answer line when you review them, and star questions that you need to review more). Try out each technique and see which works for you.

You can download Anki for free from their website (apps.ankiweb.net). Pre-made decks can be found around the net, especially on *Reddit*, with a quick Google search. Additionally, consider asking classmates and upper-semester students if they have any Anki decks made specifically for your school's exams. A valuable time saver!

➤ 3. Question banks

It is extremely important for your board exams, your general learning of medicine, and, to an extent, your school exams, that you go through question banks.

Question banks substantially deepen your understanding by making you apply knowledge in new, challenging ways, and helping you differentiate closely related things from each other. They also ensure you cover the most critical information in each subject. The very process of thinking critically about the information and getting questions wrong also helps cement it into your long-term memory.

Simply put, if you have gone through the *UWorld* question bank for a particular subject and understand/remember the majority of what you've learned from them, it's fairly safe to say you've learned the subject pretty well.

How many question banks should I go through?

> **One** during school terms, and an additional one if you have a couple of months off to study.

During your semesters, it's unlikely you will have time to go through more than one major question bank (e.g., *UWorld*, *Kaplan*, *USMLE-Rx*, etc.). But you need to do at least one! After all basic science courses are complete, some schools give students a few months off to prepare for the USMLE Step 1 (e.g., US, Caribbean schools). If you do have such a break, it's useful to go through another question bank during that time.

Choice of question banks

The gold standard for question banks is undoubtedly **UWorld**. It is highly recommended that you complete the entire *UWorld* USMLE Step 1 question bank at some point before you move on from the basic sciences. Good options for a second question bank, should you have the time to use one, include:

1. Kaplan Qbank
2. Board Vitals
3. USMLE-Rx

If you anticipate that you'll have a significant study break after you've completed your basic science courses, consider completing one of the three alternative question banks *first* and saving *UWorld* for last. While they're all quite similar, *UWorld* tends to have the most challenging questions and is thought to be the closest replica of the USMLE Step 1, which may make it most advantageous *after* you've acquired a decent proficiency of your subjects.

Keep in mind the above three question banks are significantly cheaper than *UWorld*, which is another reason why they might be great options for when you're first learning the subjects during your school semesters.

Learning efficiently from question banks

Prioritize learning over numbers

Throughout medical school, you will likely hear some students proclaiming that they go through intimidatingly large numbers of questions per day. Rest assured – the number of questions you go through per day doesn't really mean much. So, don't be unnerved by these claims and don't give them much attention. Far more important is how well you learn from them.

What is the ultimate point of doing questions? They are simply tools to teach you new things and allow you to see facts and topics in a new light. You don't learn new things by reading questions, nor by answering them – you learn new things by reading the explanations and further investigating gaps in your knowledge.

Therefore, even when you've answered a question correctly, read the explanation and ask questions. Often, you'll find you learn something valuable even for questions you felt confident with. For topics you're very familiar with, you can skim rather than read.

Ask the following three questions after seeing the answer to each question:

1. What **key features** make the correct answer correct?
2. Why exactly are the **other answer** choices wrong?
3. Were there any **details** I was unclear about?

For example, let's consider this real, retired NBME anatomy question:

A 20-year-old man is brought to the emergency department 1 hour after he was involved in a motorcycle collision. He was not wearing a helmet. Physical examination shows clear fluid dripping from the nose. X-rays show a fracture of the cribriform plate of the ethmoid bone. This patient is at greatest risk for impairment of which of the following senses?

(A) Balance
(B) Hearing
(C) Olfaction
(D) Taste from the anterior two thirds of the tongue
(E) Taste from the posterior one third of the tongue
(F) Vision

Suppose you answered this question correctly (*i.e.,* choice c – olfaction) because you know that the olfactory nerve travels through the cribriform plate. While many students might simply move on after seeing that they answered correctly, let's try the three-question strategy described above:

1. *What **key features** make the correct answer correct?*

    ➢ Great – you've understood this.

2. *Why exactly are the **other answer** choices wrong?*

    Choice A

    ➢ What nerve is responsible for balance? → vestibulocochlear nerve
    ➢ What cranial opening does that nerve come out of? → internal acoustic meatus

    Choice B, etc.

3. *Were there any **details** in the question you were unclear about?*

    ➢ *"cribriform plate of the ethmoid bone"* – did I know the cribriform plate is part of the ethmoid bone?
    ➢ *"clear fluid dripping from the nose"* – do I know what this means? (Clear fluid from the nose after head trauma signifies **cerebrospinal fluid leak**)

This method does take time, at least initially, but is well worth the effort when exam time comes!

So, focus on how *much* you're learning rather than how *many* questions you're completing.

To summarize:

1. **Reflect and ask questions,** and
2. **Always read the explanations**.

Taking notes from question banks

It is essential to take good notes of any new facts or concepts you learn while going through questions. These are the gems of the question bank, and if you don't preserve them, you'll have spent a ton of time completing questions for very little reward. Without writing them down and reviewing them, you will forget many of them.

There are two forms of notes to take:

1. **Electronic notes** (*Microsoft Word* or *Anki*).

  o This allows you to both take notes and review them rapidly.

2. **Annotating your *First Aid*** for any new concept or *worthwhile* fact.

  o This improves your *First Aid* as a reference and review book, and effectively compartmentalizes the new information.

  o Note: annotating takes time, and you don't want to flood your copy with notes, so use your judgement and leave less important facts for your electronic notes alone.

Notes can be concise facts, or you can write them as questions. Writing out facts is generally better for larger concepts, while writing questions may be better for random, isolated bits of new information. Doing this in *Microsoft Word* is generally faster than *Anki*. To do so, as described above, write out the question on one line, then write the answer in the line below it. When reviewing these questions, you can slowly scroll down so that you only see the question at first, then scroll more to reveal the answer line.

➤ 4. Commercial video series

Commercial video series are video lecture courses by various companies that teach you all major subjects of the basic sciences.

These can be extremely useful, both because they are generally high in teaching quality and because they effectively highlight the highest-yield information for board exams (namely, the USMLE Step 1) and real life. This makes them especially useful when your school's lecturer for a particular subject isn't great or their lecture content isn't well-structured (which unfortunately can be a common occurrence), or if you simply prefer learning at your own pace.

There are four top series that cover all major basic science subjects. They are (along with a sample video for each):

1. *Kaplan*
  ➤ www.youtube.com/watch?v=V69j4Apn8vI
2. *Boards and Beyond*
  ➤ www.youtube.com/watch?v=DUtyVHXbtwA
3. *Doctors In Training (DIT)*
  ➤ www.youtube.com/watch?v=mdEhC0bRJ5U
4. *Lecturio*
  ➤ www.youtube.com/watch?v=YwdYf4Yd3DE

Kaplan and **Boards and Beyond** are most commonly recognized by students as the best series, but all four are safe bets.

Subject-specific series

For a few subjects, though, there are subject-specific video series that take precedence over the aforementioned ones. They are:

! TIP

Consider listening to certain lecturers at an **increased speed**. There's a balance between speed and comprehension, so speeds between 1.25x - 1.75x usually work best. However, see what works best for you for a given lecturer and topic. Easier topics and slower speakers can be sped up more than confusing topics and fast speakers.

1. Pathology: **Pathoma** video lectures are the gold standard, and they are a MUST for studying pathology.
2. Microbiology: **Sketchy Micro** is very highly recommended.
3. Pharmacology: **Sketchy Pharm** is highly recommended.

SECTION 6

Subject Guides

What follows are guides for each major **subject** in medical school. Tips for specific **organ systems** (e.g., cardiovascular, respiratory, etc.) can be found within the relevant subject guides – namely, in anatomy, physiology, pathology, and pharmacology.

Remember that all YouTube links are listed at **dryoumethod.com/companion_links** for convenience.

1. Clinical Skills

The focus of clinical skills classes in the basic sciences is getting you prepared you for clinical rotations by acquainting you with history-taking, physical examination, and note-writing. You'll encounter most of the skills you learn again and again throughout your clinical rotations – each time becoming more proficient – so don't be disheartened if you're not feeling confident in your abilities – this is normal!

Intensity: low

Memorization: 2.5/5

Content emphasis on board exams: technical skills not applicable for theory exams; however, responses to various patient encounters and questions is **medium-high** (see *Special scenarios* on page 73).

➤ Approach & guidelines

There are three pillars of clinical skills in the basic sciences: **history-taking**, **physical examination**, and **note-writing**.

History-taking

When memorizing history questions and the order in which to ask them, it's easy to overlook how logical history-taking is actually supposed to be.

Thinking about the history purely as a checklist will cause you to make mistakes and forget things, especially under pressure (both in exams and in real life!). While there are some things you simply have to memorize, it is immensely beneficial to give a logical order to the history. To do this, think of how you would try to systematically solve a problem outside of medicine (for example, a computer issue). This can help you understand the concept of history-taking.

Think about each section of the history like this:

1. First, what's the problem? (**Chief complaint**)
2. Tell me all the details of the problem [when it started, how it started, if it's happened before, etc.] (**History of presenting illness**)
3. What problems have you had in the past? (**Past medical history**)
   a. The current problem might be related to past issues.
4. Do any family members have related issues? (**Family history**)
5. Are there any lifestyle factors that might have caused these issues? (**Social history**)
6. Let me just systematically ask a bunch of questions to make sure I didn't miss anything (**Review of systems**)

That is essentially it! The components of a generic history are:

- Chief complaint
- History of presenting illness
- Past medical/surgical history
- Medications/allergies
- Family history
- Social history
- Review of systems

In some scenarios you will also need to obtain a sexual, obstetric, pediatric, or psychiatric history.

Physical Exam

There aren't really any secrets to learning and perfecting your physical exam other than to practice abundantly, visualize things when practicing on your own, and to always **proceed from head to toe**.

By moving from head to toe, you are literally following the body of the person right in front of you, which helps you avoid missing or forgetting things. Proceeding in an arbitrary pattern requires you to stop, think and remember an abstract order, and a greater chance you might miss something. This head-to-toe sequence applies both when moving from system to system (e.g., head/neck to respiratory to cardio to abdominal, etc.) as well as when working within a system (e.g., in a cardiovascular exam, examine eyes, then neck veins/arteries, then the heart, then check legs for edema, etc.)

The major systems for a physical examination are

1. General (constitutional)
2. Head, Eyes, Ears, Nose, Throat (HEENT)
3. Respiratory
4. Cardiovascular
5. Gastrointestinal
6. Genitourinary
7. Musculoskeletal
8. Skin (integumentary)
9. Neurologic
10. Psychiatric

Under normal circumstances, you would _not_ need to examine all of these in a single physical exam – only those that are relevant to the patient in front of you; this is called a *focused examination.*

Note-writing

Note-writing is relatively simple, and compared to history-taking and physical examination, it generally requires the least amount of practice. This is because all it entails is essentially writing out what you found in your history and physical exam, and adding an assessment ("I think the patient has this or that illness") and plan ("I want to do these investigations and start this treatment"). This is what's called the standard "**SOAP note**" format (<u>S</u>ubjective, <u>O</u>bjective, <u>A</u>ssessment, <u>P</u>lan). Here is a simple summary of the SOAP note:

<u>S</u>ubjective (the history)

Subjective means *what the patient says* – in other words, the **history**. Therefore, in this section, all you need to do is write out the pertinent history in essentially the same order as you are supposed to obtain it (chief complaint, history of presenting illness, past medical history, etc.)

<u>O</u>bjective (the physical exam)

Objective means what *you* have found – in other words, your **physical exam**. Therefore, in this section, simply write out your physical exam findings, system by system. Be sure to include pertinent negative findings (e.g., no abdominal tenderness).

<u>A</u>ssessment

Assessment is simply your **diagnosis** and **differential diagnoses** (other possible diagnoses that you must consider). You may also include the urgency of the situation, if relevant. For example:

> *"23-year-old man with a past history of type 1 diabetes presenting with signs/symptoms of **diabetic ketoacidosis** and requiring urgent resuscitation.*
>
> *Differential diagnoses: alcohol withdrawal, sepsis"*

<u>P</u>lan

Plan is…your **plan**. Divide this section into investigations (e.g., imaging studies, blood tests) and treatments (e.g., start antibiotics). Write these out in bullet-point form.

Special Scenarios

Aside from the three core skills (history, physical, and notes), there is one area of clinical skills that is particularly important for all major board examinations – both theoretical and clinical: **responding to specific patient scenarios**. This ranges from handling angry patients to delivering bad news, to recognizing patients with poor health literacy.

Recurring themes in the majority of these scenarios are: **responding in an empathetic way**, **assuming responsibility**, and **protecting confidentiality**. Therefore, if you encounter such questions on an exam, give strong consideration to the most empathetic and responsible answer. Occasionally, they may try to trick you with a special situation (e.g., a patient who is asking for something unethical) in which you need to be firm and straightforward (while being respectful), so be mindful and consider the other answer choices as well. However, most of the time, the correct answer is the most empathetic, responsible, and confidentiality-respecting one.

A useful way to become skilled at handling these scenarios correctly (both in exams and real life) is to visualize a doctor you know whom you feel embodies empathetic and responsible patient care very well, and imagine how they would respond in that scenario. This can often be one of your clinical skills professors.

➤ Top resources

Your 3 top resources for clinical skills are your **school's clinical skills classes**, **YouTube** (especially for physical exams), and **Geeky Medics**.

Geeky Medics *(GeekyMedics.com)*

Geeky Medics is a website with excellent, easy-to-follow written guides for history taking and physical examination. They also have arguably the best history and physical examination videos on *YouTube*. *Geeky Medics* will be an invaluable resource for you.

Textbooks

In addition, you may choose to use a textbook. This is a personal preference (unless required by your school), so keep in mind you do not need them to succeed. Many students do excellent in clinical skills without even opening a textbook. Some, however, might simply prefer that their source of reference be a book rather than a website or YouTube videos, in which case two of the best textbooks are **Bates' Guide to Physical Examination and History Taking** (which also comes in a "pocket" edition) and **Talley & O'Connor's Clinical Examination**.

➤ Useful YouTube channels

Geeky Medics

As discussed above, Geeky Medics has arguably the best physical examination videos on YouTube.

➤ https://www.youtube.com/user/geekymedics123

Physiotutors

Physiotutors has arguably the highest-quality videos for musculoskeletal/orthopedic tests on YouTube. Refer to them for any joint-related or musculoskeletal tests, especially for the knee and shoulder (rotator cuff).

➢ https://www.youtube.com/user/Physiotutors

➢ **Useful YouTube videos & series**

How I ranked 1ˢᵗ in Cambridge University | Medical History Taking Approach [Arun Kiru]

A great and concise walkthrough of taking an effective patient history.

➢ https://www.youtube.com/watch?v=vGTzlCIaD3Y

➢ **Tips & key concepts**

Taking Pauses

During OSCE examinations, be comfortable with simply **taking pauses** when you need to think about the next history question or physical exam maneuver. It might feel uncomfortable initially, but in reality, there's nothing awkward about it. It looks much better and more confident than saying lots of "ummm"s or looking frantic.

More importantly though, having a calm pause allows you to think a lot better than when you're nervously keeping conversation going or scrambling to proceed to the next question or maneuver. Just pause, relax, and think calmly. If you feel more comfortable, you can even give the examiner and the standardized patient a heads-up by having a prepared phrase for such pauses, like "Just a moment, if you don't mind".

Open-ended Questions

Remember to start off your history by asking general, **open-ended questions**. Allow the patient to tell their story! Not only is this a more thorough approach, but it also makes your job so much easier. Remember to ask, "Anything else?" After letting the patient tell their story, *then* fill in the gaps by asking more specific, closed-ended questions (e.g., have you had any fever?).

Standard Introduction

Engrave into your routine for every single history-taking and physical examination the standard introduction. These are simple things that you'll always need to say/do and that will score you a few free points on every OSCE exam without any thought. These are:

1. Knock on the door
2. Sanitize hands
3. Greet patient and explain who you are
4. Describe what you plan to do and ask for permission
5. Confirm name and age (or date of birth)

NOTES

2. Anatomy

Anatomy is one of the most valuable introductory subjects in the basic sciences because it helps you to understand many pathologies. Furthermore, anatomy is widely applicable across medical specialties. Unlike some subjects that might not be too useful for the particular specialty you're interested in, strong knowledge in anatomy will benefit you in almost every specialty.

Intensity: high

Memorization: 5/5

Content emphasis on board exams: medium

Only very rarely will you see a question on a major board exam (USMLE, MCCQE, etc.) that simply asks you to identify such and such structure. There are many questions, however, that either test the clinical anatomy, i.e., related to a disease or injury (e.g., brachial plexus injury syndromes, common areas where nerves are injured, the anatomy around hernias, etc.) or test knowledge of anatomy that is important to understanding the disease.

➤ Approach & guidelines

Repetition

Anatomy is one of, if not, the most memorization-heavy subject in all of medicine. As such, there is simply no way around repetition. You need to encounter and test yourself on the information at least a few times to solidify it into your memory. It also helps to look at and feel *real life* anatomy, such as in the dissection room, and to relate your knowledge to your own day-to-day activities – e.g., "which muscles am I using now?"

Pattern Recognition

While anatomy is memorization-heavy, this *does not* mean you should only aim to memorize information as scattered facts. One of the most useful techniques is to find patterns in the information. These help to both understand *and* remember anatomy. The patterns are often found in the names of structures, i.e., in the etymology, or root words. It pays to become acquainted with some of the more common Latin and Greek root words!

Some important patterns to look for include:

- The name can reflect a structure's:
  - Location: The region of the body in which it is located, e.g., the name of the **supraspinatus** muscle tells you that it lies **above** the **spine** of the scapula

- o Appearance or qualities: e.g., a **circ**umflex artery tells you it **circles** around a structure.
- o Attachments: Muscles with two-part names that tell you its origin and insertion, e.g., the **hyoglossus** muscle originates from the **hyoid** bone and attaches to the **tongue** (**glossus**)

- All the muscles within a muscle **compartment** usually have the same innervation and blood supply.
- Superficial **muscle layers** are generally larger and act on larger, proximal joints, while deep muscle layers are generally smaller and act on smaller, distal joints.
- Patterns in the **layers** of structures, e.g., the abdominal wall is essentially a sandwich around muscle, with fascia, fat, and a thin additional layer around it on each side, in that order.
- Patterns in **numbering**, e.g., the cranial nerves are numbered in the order that they emerge from the brain/brainstem; the 8 liver segments are numbered in a clockwise fashion (looking from head on).
- Patterns in **size, location, or appearance**, e.g., the **medial** cerebellum helps with coordination of **medial** parts of the body (i.e., the trunk, proximal limbs), while the **lateral** cerebellum helps with coordination of **lateral** parts of the body (i.e., extremities).

You may well be amazed by how many patterns there are in the information if you invest a little time into reflecting on it.

First Learn the Bare Skeleton

When first learning an anatomical part, it's very important (and time efficient) to start by developing a very clear mental image of the part. In other words, in the beginning, you need to break the part down to its absolute skeleton and filter out any additional details. Think of it as a jigsaw puzzle: rather than starting off randomly assembling various pieces here and there, you need to get a clear, simple mental picture of it at its most basic level and know what its main features are (e.g., a sunset, a mountain, and a lake).

For example, the lower extremity has many arteries with numerous branches, which can make learning them a bit overwhelming at first. However, by breaking it down to its bare skeleton, you may find it significantly easier to digest. That skeleton is:

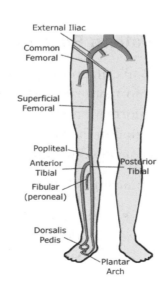

- The **external iliac** artery goes down the leg and experiences three name changes, becoming the **common femoral**, **superficial femoral**, and **popliteal** arteries.
- At the knee, the popliteal artery divides into 3 – the **anterior tibial**, **posterior tibial**, and **fibular** arteries.
- The anterior tibial artery becomes the **dorsalis pedis** artery, the **posterior tibial** artery becomes the **plantar arch**, and the two systems anastomose in the foot.

That's it!

Image Search

To help you get that bare skeleton, this is where your good friend *Google Images* comes in. A Google search will turn up tons of images of the given structure – some extremely detailed and others very basic. Learn from the basic ones *first*. Once you've developed a clear understanding and mental image of the structure, you can then start to learn the finer details. Those details will now be much more neatly organized in your mind and will be integrated as part of a larger picture.

> **TIP**
>
> Try and **avoid long "phrase" mnemonics** (e.g. *Some Angry Lady Figured Out PMS*). Though they can initially feel helpful, by the end of your course your actual anatomical understanding will be foggy.

➤ Top resources

Google Images and **YouTube** are *especially* valuable for anatomy given how visual the subject is. Additionally, remember to check the anatomy section at the beginning of each organ system in your *First Aid* book. While these sections are very brief, what they do contain is generally quite important and well-presented.

In addition, some useful resources are listed below. These are options to consider for making your studies easier and more efficient. Don't *overdo* the resources though– you DO NOT need all of these to succeed in anatomy.

Textbooks

Fire Anatomy Mnemonics

Though written by myself(!), all promotion aside, the book *Fire Anatomy Mnemonics* does genuinely have a lot of very useful mnemonics and explanations that will likely save you a lot of time in studying. It is not a primary resource in the sense that it does not cover every single thing in anatomy, but it is very useful as a supplementary resource to help you save time and make life a little easier. It is highly visual with lots of clear and memorable images.

Netter's Atlas of Human Anatomy

Owning a full-length anatomy textbook is likely unnecessary. With such a vast array of images and videos available on the internet for free, these books are more a matter of personal preference/ enjoyment. If you do opt for a textbook as a primary source, your top choice might be **Netter's Atlas of Human Anatomy**. This is a big book with lots of quality drawings of different anatomical regions and organs. Flick through it in the library or use Amazon's *Look Inside*

> **TIP**
>
> Unless required, avoid buying the textbook *Grant's Dissector*. It mainly just teaches you cadaveric dissection techniques, which makes it unuseful outside of your school's dissection classes.

feature to view its content and see if you like it.

Question banks (paid)

BRS Gross Anatomy

If your library has the textbook **BRS Gross Anatomy,** or if you don't mind spending a few dollars to buy it (it's cheap), doing the questions at the end of each chapter can be very helpful. The questions are short and not too difficult, which may be more advantageous and time-efficient when first learning anatomy than long "UWorld-style" questions. They test important concepts, including clinical correlates, and help ensure you're adequately learning the bread and butter of the subject.

USMLE Question Banks

If you're returning to anatomy for review, USMLE step 1 question banks (**UWorld**, **Kaplan**, etc.) are critical, as they'll ensure you're on top of the most clinically relevant correlates. If learning anatomy for the first time, these question banks may also be useful if you have spare time after going through a simpler question bank (e.g., BRS Gross Anatomy). Keep in mind, however, that UWorld questions are generally quite challenging and might touch on some things beyond the scope of your school's anatomy exams.

Question banks (free)

The benefit of the BRS Gross Anatomy questions is that you can be certain all the questions are highly clinically relevant and geared towards the major board exams (most notably the USMLE Step 1). However, there are two free online question banks which can still be excellent sources of practice questions and are worthwhile to consider using – these are **BlueLink: University of Michigan** and **Texas Tech University Anatomy Questions**. Both are very clinically oriented.

BlueLink: University of Michigan

➢ *https://sites.google.com/a/umich.edu/bluelink/resources/practice-questions*

Texas Tech University Anatomy Questions

➢ *https://anatomy.elpaso.ttuhsc.edu/musculoskeletal_system/thigh_questions.html*

Websites

KenHub (KenHub.com)

In terms of the quality of images, **KenHub** has some of the best and clearest images you'll find on the internet. They highlight the relevant anatomical part in a deep green color that makes the image both exceptionally clear and memorable. You can find their images with a search on Google Images and clicking on them takes you to a well-organized explanation of the part.

These articles are free, though KenHub has some other features like video tutorials and quizzes that require a paid subscription.

TeachMeAnatomy (TeachMeAnatomy.info/subjects)

TeachMeAnatomy is similar to KenHub in that they have lots of free breakdowns of anatomical regions/topics. The advantage of TeachMeAnatomy is that their explanations are simpler and clearer, and they focus mostly on the essentials. They also present high-yield clinical correlates in big black boxes. If you don't use the site for anything else, it might be worth it just to run through every topic and review the *Clinical Significance* box, as these are really meaningful.

➤ Useful YouTube channels

AnatomyZone

This channel uses a neat simulation program to demonstrate anatomy and explains concepts very clearly. On their website, they have high-quality interactive 3D models for some body parts as well (www.AnatomyZone.com).

➤ https://www.youtube.com/user/TheAnatomyZone

Institute of Human Anatomy

This channel uses high-quality cadavers to demonstrate interesting or important anatomical concepts in very engaging ways, including clinical correlates. While it might not teach you the bread and butter of anatomy, what it does teach you can really deepen your understanding of the subject and will likely be remembered very well, given how fascinating the illustrations are.

➤ https://www.youtube.com/channel/UCgBg0aacyJnw4qUnb1FlfEQ

Sam Webster

Sam Webster simply does an excellent job explaining anatomy using plastic anatomical models (which are surprisingly effective!). In particular, check out his 'Popular Uploads' section, as some of his best videos have the most views.

➤ https://www.youtube.com/c/SamWebster

➤ Useful YouTube videos & series

Autonomic Nerves of the Abdomen [James Pickering]

The autonomic innervation of the abdomen is a very confusing topic that can take a long time to grasp, and this 11-minute video presents it exceptionally well.

➤ https://www.youtube.com/watch?v=WXO_nyFY9oM

How to Remember the Cranial Nerves [karthik bhandari]

A great system of mnemonics to remember the cranial nerves using your fingers. This is very effective as using your fingers makes it easy to remember them during an exam. Bear in mind the mistake involving cranial nerve 4 – it actually *depresses*, *abducts*, and *intorts* the eye.

➢   https://www.youtube.com/watch?v=kqNFmBGHs2I

An easy way to remember arm muscles [marfi0904]

Two videos that make learning all the muscles of the arm and forearm very simple. Possibly two of the most valuable anatomy videos on the internet, these videos are a must-see.

➢   Part 1: https://www.youtube.com/watch?v=iDXUwErttJA&t=199s
➢   Part 2: https://www.youtube.com/watch?v=qomVodg-5SM&t=194s

---

> ➢   **Tips & key concepts**

Pay particular attention to anatomical parts and concepts that relate to clinical syndromes, as these are both favorite topics for exam questions and important knowledge for practicing real medicine. The following are some of these "can't-miss" topics. See the book *Fire Anatomy Mnemonics* for more mnemonics and tricks.

General

Parietal vs. Visceral

There are three main cavities that are lined by "parietal" and "visceral" layers: the **pericardium**, **lung pleura**, and **abdominal cavity**. Substances (fluid or air) can accumulate between these two layers, causing compression of the underlying organ (cardiac tamponade in the heart, pneumothorax/pleural effusion in the lung, and abdominal compartment syndrome in the abdomen).

  o   Think: the *parietal* layer is the *parent* – it covers/protects the inner visceral layer.

Arteries and Veins

- Uterine artery vs. ureter: "*water* flows *under* the *bridge*"
  o   The **ureter** (water) passes under the **uterine artery** (bridge)
  o   Important because the ureter may be mistaken for the uterine artery during surgery and accidentally ligated, leading to an obstructed ureter.
- Left vs. right gonadal vein:
  o   The right gonadal vein drains directly into the IVC, while the left gonadal vein first drains into the left renal vein.
  o   The IVC is on the right side of the body, so naturally the left gonadal vein has to travel further to reach it. Alternatively, think: Left = Longer path.

  - This is important since the left gonadal vein enters the left renal vein at a 90-degree angle, making flow less laminar and hence higher in pressure in the left gonadal vein. This is why **varicocele** (swollen veins inside the scrotum) is **more common on the left**.
- Infection in the face can spread to the cavernous sinus because the **facial vein** anastomoses with the **superior ophthalmic veins**. This can lead to **cavernous sinus thrombosis.**

Cardiovascular

The **left atrium** is the most posterior chamber of the heart.

- Clinical correlate: Directly behind the left atrium lies the **esophagus**. Enlargement of the left atrium can compress the esophagus, causing dysphagia (difficulty swallowing).
- Think: the **LA** is the **LA**st part of the heart before the esophagus

Gastrointestinal

Porto-systemic anastomoses

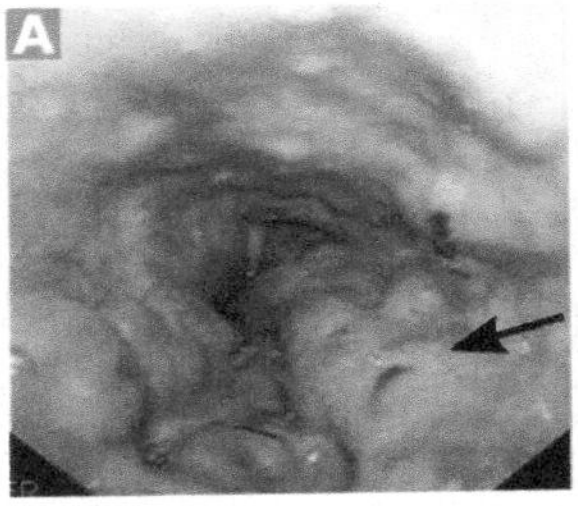

Porto-systemic anastomoses are where the portal venous system meets the systemic venous system. These are important because liver disease causes backflow and increased pressure in the portal circulation. This opens up these anastomoses and causes venous dilation.

In the esophagus, these dilations are called **esophageal varices** A. These can rupture and cause life-threatening hemorrhage. The three important porto-systemic anastomoses are:

1. *Esophagus*: Between **left gastric** (portal) and **azygos** (systemic) veins.
2. *Rectum*: Between **superior rectal** (portal) and middle/**inferior rectal** (systemic) veins.
3. *Umbilicus*: Between **paraumbilical** (portal) and **small epigastric** (systemic) veins.

Intraperitoneal vs. Retroperitoneal Organs

Knowing intraperitoneal vs. retroperitoneal organs is extremely clinically important for a *ton* of reasons. The retroperitoneal organs are: **SADPUCKER**

1. **S**: suprarenal (adrenal) gland
2. **A**: aorta/IVC
3. **D**: duodenum (2nd & 3rd part)
4. **P**: pancreas (except tail)
5. **U**: ureters
6. **C**: colon (ascending & descending)
7. **K**: kidneys
8. **E**: esophagus
9. **R**: rectum

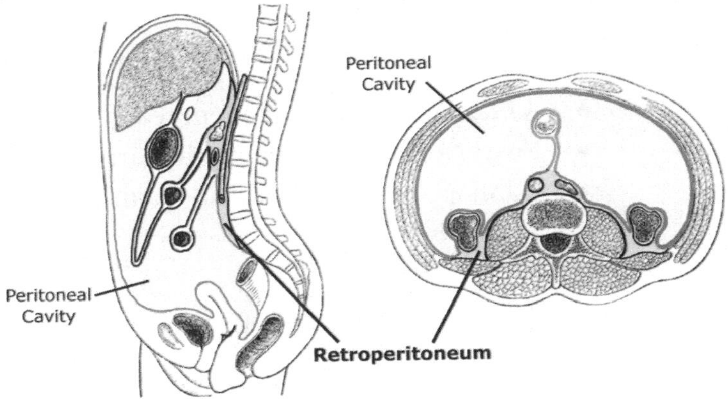

Inguinal Hernias

- **Direct** inguinal hernias push **directly** through the abdominal wall; *medial* to the inferior epigastric artery.
- **In**direct inguinal hernias travel **in** the **in**guinal canal; *lateral* to the inferior epigastric artery.

Most Dependent Parts of the Abdomen

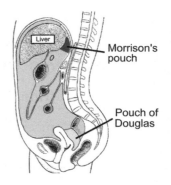

- When upright: **pouch of** Douglas (females only)
  - Think: the deepest hole that can be **dug**
- When supine: **Morrison's pouch**

Pancreas

- The tail of the pancreas *tickles* the spleen (i.e., the spleen lies at the tip of the pancreatic tail).
  - Clinical correlate: An inflamed pancreas (pancreatitis) can spread its inflammation to the adjacent splenic vein, leading to **splenic vein thrombosis.**

Musculoskeletal

Common spots for nerve injury

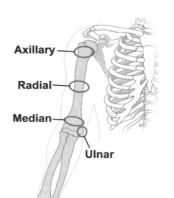

- Arm
  - Surgical head of humerus fracture: **Axillary nerve**
  - Mid-shaft of humerus fracture: **Radial nerve**
  - Supracondylar fracture: **Median nerve**
  - Medial epicondylar fracture: **Ulnar nerve**
- Leg
  - Fibular head: **Common peroneal nerve**

Median Nerve

Know the median nerve's sensory and motor innervation (examiners love testing this because it relates to **carpal tunnel syndrome**).

Knee Ligaments

Ligaments of the knee and associated physical exam tests:

- **Anterior** cruciate ligament tear: **Anterior** drawer test.
- **Posterior** cruciate ligament tear: **Posterior** drawer test.
- "Unhappy triad": ACL, MCL, and medial meniscus injury from lateral blow to knee.

Neurovascular Bundles

The order of structures in neurovascular bundles is frequently tested because they're important to know to be able to safely obtain intravascular access, perform procedures, etc.

- Femoral triangle *(lateral to medial)*: **N**erve, **A**rtery, **V**ein ("**NAV**y").
- Cubital fossa contents *(lateral to medial)*: **T**endon [of biceps], **A**rtery [brachial], **N**erve [median] ("**TAN**").
- Intercostal nerves and vessels *(superior to inferior)*: **V**ein, **A**rtery, **N**erve ("**VAN**").

Serratus Anterior

The serratus anterior is innervated by the **long thoracic nerve**. Injury to the nerve causes the CLASSIC "**winged scapula**" 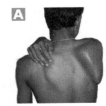. The second you hear "*winged scapula*", think long thoracic nerve injury.

Rotator Cuff

The four muscles are ("**SITS**"):

1. Supraspinatus
2. Infraspinatus
3. Teres minor
4. Subscapularis

Remember the functions of each muscle by knowing the general location of each, and then remembering that all four insert onto the lateral part of the humerus. Once you remember the functions, the physical exam maneuvers are not hard to remember, as they simply test that function.

Functions and tests:

- **Supraspinatus** *(abduction)*: Empty Can test, Drop Arm test
  - Clinical correlate: Supraspinatus is the most commonly injured rotator cuff muscle, so if you have to guess, choose "supraspinatus".
- **Infraspinatus** and **teres minor** *(external rotation)*: simple external rotation.
- **Subscapularis** *(internal rotation)*: Lift Off test, Bear-hug test.
  - Remember: *subscapularis* is the only one on the anterior side of the scapula, and hence the only one that internally rotates the arm.
- Other: **impingement syndrome** is tested for by Neer's test.

Ligamentum Flavum

The **ligamentum flavum** is the last spinal ligament before the epidural space – the space you access in epidural anesthesia (think: the ligamentum *flavum* can literally taste the **flavor** of the epidural space). When you penetrate the ligament, you feel a "pop".

Trendelenburg sign

Trendelenburg sign is when a lesion to the **superior** **gluteal nerve** causes the *contralateral* side of the hip to sag because of a weakened **gluteus medius** and **minimus**.

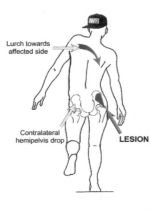

o <u>Think</u>: a **Trend**y new way to walk for those who feel **superior**.

Scaphoid

The **scaphoid** is the most commonly injured carpal bone. It gets injured by a fall on an outstretched hand, resulting in pain in the **anatomical snuff box**. Fracture can lead to **avascular necrosis** of the scaphoid due to its retrograde blood flow.

Neurology

Layers of the meninges

- **Dura**: **dura**ble, outermost layer.
- **Arachnoid**: **spider web**-like connections that absorb CSF (*arachnoid* means *spider*).
- **Pia**: delicate, innermost layer that adheres to the brain and spinal cord like the delicate crust of a **pie.**

Cranial Nerves

Know ALL cranial nerves as they are <u>super</u> important for both exams and clinical medicine (e.g., injured by certain strokes, tumors, neuropathies etc.).

Cranial nerve	Function	Mnemonic
1: Olfactory	Smell (olfaction)	Pick your **nose** with **1** finger.
2: Optic	Sight	Make the "I'm **watching you**" sign with **2** fingers.
3: Oculomotor	Eye movement (all ocular muscles except superior oblique and lateral rectus) Eyelid opening Pupillary constriction Accommodation	Make the "OK" sign with **3** fingers over both eyes to keep your eyelids open (**eyelid opening**), look around through the holes (***most eye movement muscles***), and squeeze your eyeball (**pupillary constriction, accommodation**).
4: Trochlear	Eye depression and intortion (via superior oblique muscle)	*"CN 4: eyes to the floor"*

5: Trigeminal	Facial sensation (ophthalmic, maxillary, and mandibular divisions) Mastication Anterior 2/3 of tongue sensation	Wipe your **face** and **eat** with your hand (each done with **5** fingers)
6: Abducens	Eye abduction (via lateral rectus muscle)	*"CN 6 makes your eyes do the splits"*
7: Facial	Facial expression muscles Lacrimation Salivation Eyelid closing Auditory volume modulation (via stapedius muscle) Taste from anterior 2/3 of tongue	Picture someone terrified and crying in fear of the **7** deadly sins (= **facial expression muscles**, **lacrimation**, **salivation**). They're closing their eyes in fear (**eyelid closing**) and plugging their ears (**auditory volume modulation**).
8: Vestibulocochlear	Hearing Balance	Make the "I can't **hear** you" sign with 4 fingers from each hand (4 + 4 = **8**).
9: Glossopharyngeal	Swallowing Elevation of pharynx/larynx (stylopharyngeus muscle) Posterior 1/3 of tongue taste and sensation Carotid body and baroreceptor/chemoreceptor innervation Salivation (parotid gland)	As its name implies, the **glosso-pharyngeal** is all about the throat (the **pharynx**) and the (back of the) tongue (the **glossus**). Simply think of all the functions that relate to these areas. Picture a fish hook (looks like a **9**) getting stuck in a person's **throat**.
10: Vagus	Parasympathetics (to thoracic and abdominal organs) Swallowing Soft palate elevation Cough reflex Talking Monitoring aortic arch baro-/chemoreceptors Keeping uvula midline	Remember the **vagus** nerve supplying **parasympathetics** by thinking of a "**relaxing** vacation in **Vegas**". **Vagus** nerve keeps the u**V**ula midline.
11: Accessory	Trapezius (shrugging) and sternocleidomastoid (head rotation) innervation	The trapezius and sternocleidomastoid muscles look like the number **11**. ▣ Trapezius ▣ SCM
12: Hypoglossal	Tongue movement	The **last** cranial nerve is for **language**.

Conus medullaris vs. Cauda equina

These two are important to differentiate because each has its own distinct syndrome when injured:

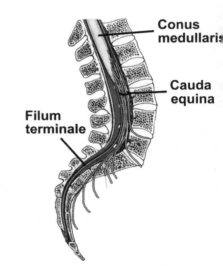

- **Conus medullaris:** part of the **spinal cord** (it's simply the *cone* at the spinal cord's bottom end). Hence, conus medullaris syndrome produces **upper** motor neuron lesion signs.
- **Cauda equina:** NOT part of the spinal cord but rather a collection of **peripheral nerves** that come off the conus medullaris like a *horse's tail* (cauda equina literally means *horse's tail*). Hence, cauda equina syndrome produces **lower** motor neuron lesion signs.

Epidural hematomas

Epidural hematomas are caused by injury to the **middle meningeal artery**.

Reproductive

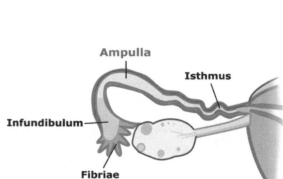

The most common site of fertilization is the **ampulla** of the fallopian tube.

- o Think: pregnancy gets **amped** up in the **ampulla**.

Respiratory

Bronchi

The **right** main bronchus is wider and more vertical than the left. Hence, inhaled foreign bodies usually end up in the right lung.

- o Think: inhaled objects go **right** down the **right** bronchus.

3. Embryology

Embryology is the study of how the embryo thingy grows and becomes a person thingy. It's important to a physician because it helps them pass medical school…

<u>Intensity:</u> low-medium

<u>Memorization:</u> 4.5/5

<u>Content emphasis on board exams:</u> *very* low

➤ Approach & guidelines

Given how low-yield embryology is for board examinations (*very* low for USMLE Step 1; essentially non-existent for MCCQE 1 and PLAB) and for practicing medicine in general, your priority should be simply to pass your school course.

In other words, place greater emphasis on what your professor wants you to know: your class lectures and handouts. Given how memorization-heavy embryology is, if you're going to be writing the USMLE Step 1 in the distant future (> 6 months), you will likely forget most of it by then anyways. Therefore, **don't spend more time on embryology than you need to**, and review the material as close to your exam as is feasible.

There are two main parts to learning embryology:

1. **Understanding/visualizing** the actual developmental process, and
2. **Memorizing** the derivatives of important structures.

Ideally, learning the developmental process more thoroughly helps you understand and memorize the important derivatives. However, this is a tradeoff, as you have limited time in medical school and embryology, as we discussed, is low yield.

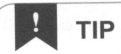

TIP

Embryology is complex and requires a lot of **visualization**. It therefore helps to see images and videos of an embryologic process from a variety of perspectives. A new perspective may often clarify a concept that is simply not making sense.

Therefore, a useful strategy is to learn and understand the major buzzwords and concepts (e.g., ectoderm/mesoderm/endoderm, neural crest, notochord, etc.) so that you have a rough idea of what the thing is, and then simply memorize the derivatives of important structures. Some of the highest yield embryology derivatives and processes (especially for the heart) are found in your *First Aid* book at the beginning of each organ system chapter.

By far most important is to learn the **clinical syndromes** and **disorders**. Other key processes and concepts you should have a basic understanding of are:

- Fertilization/implantation.
- Gastrulation (ectoderm, mesoderm, endoderm).
- Neural crest cell derivatives.
- Branchial (pharyngeal) apparatus (especially remember: DiGeorge syndrome → 3rd/4th branchial pouch defect).
- Aortic arch derivatives.
- Fetal circulation (umbilical cord parts; the 3 fetal shunts; PDA-closing/opening drugs [indomethacin → close; prostaglandins E_1 and E_2 → open]).
- Heart septum (namely as it relates to patent foramen ovale vs. septal defects).
- Thyroglossal duct.

➤ Top resources

YouTube and **Wikipedia** are two excellent resources for embryology. It usually isn't worth your time or money to get or even use an embryology textbook. Instead, it's usually more valuable to spend your time just getting a decent general conceptualization and learning high-yield facts rather than to go word-for-word through a textbook and try to pick up all the minute details. Do this by following along with the topics of your class lectures with YouTube and Wikipedia to get higher-quality explanations. If possible, pre-watch the YouTube videos referenced in *Useful YouTube videos and series,* below.

TeachMeAnatomy (www.teachmeanatomy.info/the-basics/embryology)

TeachMeAnatomy's embryology section does a nice job of explaining embryologic topics *concisely* as well as highlighting clinical correlates. Even if you're not planning on using it as a main resource, it may be worth it to simply go article-by-article and read only the **clinical correlates**, as those are by far the most important part of embryology.

➤ Useful YouTube videos & series

Series: Embryology [About Medicine]

Four videos with crisp explanations and exceptional visual representations of very confusing early embryonic concepts (1. Amniotic Cavity and Yolk Sac, 2. The First Three Weeks, 3. Neurulation, 4. Gastrulation).

➤ https://www.youtube.com/playlist?list=PL33iTqJPcF_hCIzVMMKUGPtSxpn_Cu2T2

Series: Embryology – USMLE Prep Video Course [Lecturio Medical]

A series of 10 videos explaining high-yield embryology concepts for the USMLE, including heart, spinal cord, and gastrointestinal development, as well as clinical correlates.

➤ https://www.youtube.com/playlist?list=PLVnjTkEwv-uPSnFN8DrUuWXtmqfnp-zwO

Embryology – Neurulation [Armando Hasudungan]

Neurulation (neural tube formation [the precursor to the CNS]) made simple.

➤ https://www.youtube.com/watch?v=vvBBFOu9h1w&t=8s

The Placenta: Its Development and Function [Bethea Medical Media]

A great 4-minute animation of the process of placenta formation.

➤ https://www.youtube.com/watch?v=xdibmSCNy6c

Pharyngeal Arches and its Derivatives – MASTER pharyngeal arches in LESS than 7 minutes ONLY! [DentalManiaK]

A clear explanation of the pharyngeal arches in just over 6 minutes (the pharyngeal arches are high-yield for embryology).

➤ https://www.youtube.com/watch?v=QVX3avCg7G8

Development of the Heart (3D) [Hyeonjoo Kim]

A stunning and clear 1-minute animation of heart development to help you understand this very confusing process (*highly recommended*).

➤ https://www.youtube.com/watch?v=a0qyagIgBPw

Development of the Face and Palate [Osmosis]

An outstanding 8-minute video explaining the development of the face and palate – in typical exceptional-quality Osmosis fashion.

➤ https://www.youtube.com/watch?v=iLbqzTlZ6yA

Development of the Tongue [Osmosis]

Just like the abovementioned Osmosis video, but for the tongue.

➤ https://www.youtube.com/watch?v=NzLySYOBjRY_

Medical embryology – Difficult concepts of early development [Peter J Ward]

Brilliant explanations by an exceptional teacher. The comment section alone should tell you how useful students have found this video.

➤ https://www.youtube.com/watch?v=rN3lep6roRI&t=929s

> **Tips & key concepts**

The three layers of the gut

The gut develops as 3 layers: the foregut, midgut, and hindgut. These correspond to the 3 major abdominal aortic arteries in the adult. In other words, the foregut is supplied by the celiac artery, the midgut by the superior mesenteric artery, and the hindgut by the inferior mesenteric artery.

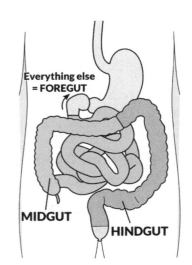

1. **Foregut**: gives rise to the esophagus, stomach, liver, gallbladder, bile ducts, pancreas, and upper duodenum.
2. **Midgut**: gives rise to everything from the lower duodenum to the proximal 2/3rds of the transverse colon.
3. **Hindgut**: gives rise to everything from the distal 1/3rd of the transverse colon to the upper anal canal.

Branchial apparatus derivatives

- Branchial apparatus derivatives: "a **CAP** covers from outside to inside".
  - **Clefts**: ectoderm
  - **Arches**: mesoderm and neural crest
  - **Pouches**: endoderm
- Branchial arch **four** gives rise to the **aorta**.
  - Think: Pronounce aorta as "**Faor**-ta"

Weeks 2, 3, and 4 of development

- Week **Two**: **Bi**laminar germ disc
- Week **Three**: **Tri**laminar germ disc
- Week **Four**: **Four** limbs appear and **Four** heart chambers (i.e., heart) start beating.

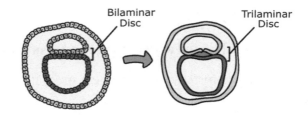

Teratogenesis

- Teratogenesis is most likely during organogenesis – between weeks three and eight
  - Think: TEratogenesis → weeks Three to Eight.

Genital development

- **Wolffian duct**: develops into **male** internal reproductive structures (think: **men** can be vicious like **wolves**).
- **Müllerian duct**: develops into female internal reproductive structures (just think of this

as "the other one").

Epispadias vs. hypospadias

Differentiate these as problems above vs. below the penis, respectively.

- **Epispadias**: bladder exstrophy
    - Epispadias is an abnormal opening along the **upper** side of the penis, hence there ought to be more associated defects *superiorly*.

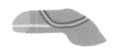

- **Hypospadias**: inguinal hernia, cryptorchidism
    - Hypospadias is an abnormal opening along the **bottom** side of the penis, hence there ought to be more associated defects *inferiorly* (the testes are located below the penis, and inguinal hernias frequently enter the scrotal sac).

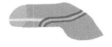

Median vs. medial umbilical ligaments

Remember that there are only two main types of fluid that must be exchanged between mom and fetus in utero: **blood** (via the umbilical vessels) and **urine** (via the urachus). These both obviously pass through the *umbilical cord*, hence when they involute, they become the *umbilical ligaments*. Remember which is which using the following logic:

- *Median* umbilical ligament: remnant of the **urachus**
    - *Median* means *"in the midline"*, which tells you there can be only *one* of it. It thus makes sense that it contains the urachus (fetus only has one urachus, just like we have only one urethra!)
- *Medial* umbilical ligaments: remnants of the **umbilical arteries**
    - *Medial* just means *"towards the midline"*, which tells you there must be *two* - one on each side of the midline. It thus makes sense that they correspond to the two umbilical arteries.

NOTES

4. Histology

Histology is the microscopic study of cells and tissues.

In medical school, the subject's main utility is to help you better understand and interpret diseases and their histological findings when you're learning pathology. If you're not going to be a pathologist, the subject's main utility to you *as a physician* is simply improving your understanding of certain disease processes. Outside of pathologists, most physicians are not tasked with interpreting histology specimens.

Intensity: low-medium

Memorization: 2/5

Content emphasis on board exams: low

! TIP

If you're reading this book purely to revise for the USMLE Step 1, you can skip this Histology chapter. You generally don't need to review histology in isolation - only as it relates to pathology.

> ❯ **Approach & guidelines**

Even more so than gross anatomy, histology is very rarely, if ever, tested on major medical board exams like the USMLE Step 1 *on its own*. In other words, questions will not simply ask you to identify a normal structure on a histology slide – rather, it will generally be applied to some pathology. For example, you might be shown a slide of neurons with classic intracellular inclusion bodies and be asked what neurodegenerative disorder this represents.

This means once you've completed your histology course and have gotten a reasonable grasp of the subject, you do NOT need to do a top-to-bottom histology review for major board exams. Most of the histological abnormalities you need to recognize are taught in pathology, so don't waste your time revisiting all of histology again.

Pattern recognition

Visual pattern recognition is central to histology. It is therefore key to view lots of histology slides. This makes Anki a particularly useful tool for histology. As you flip through slides, look to develop a good "eye" for the following two things:

1. **Understand the structures/features within a specific tissue.**

    o Especially look for unique-looking structures or organelles. Be sure to read labels and explanations.

1. **Tell organs/tissues apart from each other.**

    o Save this for the end of your exam preparation, as you need to learn the tissue-specific histology first. When you're ready, flip through a large deck of slides (e.g., using Anki) mixed together from various tissues and simply try to guess what the tissue is. This quickly improves your histology pattern recognition skills. Try to have fun with it!

If you're simply preparing for a block exam rather than your final exam, you have a few options for getting an Anki deck:

1. Download a pre-made deck from Reddit that's organized by system and select only the systems you've covered in your block.
2. Ask around to see if any of your peers (or past students) have already made a deck for that block.
3. Compile the images and make the deck yourself (last option!).

In general, it's probably not worth your time to make your own Anki histology deck. There are some great pre-made ones available on Reddit that will save you a ton of time – just do a quick Google search (e.g., "histology Anki decks").

Emphasize general principles

When it comes to preparing for board exams in particular, pay close attention to **general principles** in interpreting histology slides. You might forget specific facts like, for example, all the different layers of the epidermis, and the consequences will be pretty minimal. In contrast, understanding general principles (e.g., large, dark nuclei representing immature cells or empty, white balls represent lipid droplets) will come back to help you time and time again in pathology questions.

➤ Top resources

Additional resources (outside of YouTube, Google Images, First Aid, and Anki) are far less critical for histology than for other courses given the fact that likely won't need to return to the subject in isolation when reviewing for board exams. Therefore, don't overdo the resources!

With that said, there are still a few resources you can consider to assist you along the way:

Websites

Blue Histology (lecannabiculteur.free.fr/SITES/UNIV%20W.AUSTRALIA/mb140/Lectures.htm)

Blue Histology is a valuable free online histology guide to use as an alternative to your school lectures and slides if they're not very good. The site also has useful quizzes, however this feature currently seems to be having some issues. Regardless, you can still access the quizzes via archive.org:

➤ https://web.archive.org/web/20200701054442/https://www.lab.anhb.uwa.edu.au/mb140

Histology Guide (histologyguide.com)

Another free online resource similar to Blue Histology is **Histology Guide**. This site has exceptional images and image-viewing features like ultra-zooming and click-and-drag, and also has quizzes for some but not all topics.

Books

BRS Histology

If your course lectures and slides are terrible, a *potentially* useful review book may be **BRS Cell Biology and Histology**. Again, given how low-yield histology is, it is arguably not worth it to purchase, but it may be useful to flip through if your school library has it. An advantage of the book is that it covers all the main topics and presents the information in a concise fashion, with focus on USMLE Step 1 preparation specifically. It also has useful end-of-chapter quizzes.

> **Useful YouTube videos & series**

Series: Histology Explained for Beginners [Corporis]

A series of 8 videos that provides excellent overviews of the major systems in histology in a very clear and visually appealing fashion.

➤ https://www.youtube.com/playlist?list=PL2rpvfNeooNHjnQSPIEf9iajPFv8oNuPQ

Series: Histology – USMLE Prep Videos | Lecturio [Lecturio]

A series of 38 histology videos. Although it's not the entire Lecturio histology course, it does cover a ton of topics and can be helpful in the areas it does cover. The lecturer does speak a bit slowly, so consider playing them at x1.25 or x1.5 speed.

➤ https://www.youtube.com/playlist?list=PLVnjTkEwv-uP09IajjtqyC-tjidKRyUop

The Integumentary System, Part 1 – Skin Deep: Crash Course A&P #6 [CrashCourse]

Fun, high-quality crash course in the skin (part 1) in under 10 minutes, including layers, cell types, clinical correlates, etc.

➤ https://www.youtube.com/watch?v=Orumw-PyNjw

The Integumentary System, Part 2 – Skin Deeper: Crash Course A&P #7 [CrashCourse]

Part 2 of the previous video.

➤ https://www.youtube.com/watch?v=EN-x-zXXVwQ

Help with Histology [ThePenguinProf]

Lays out a neat dichotomous key for identifying any tissue based on physical appearance.

➢ https://www.youtube.com/watch?v=ux9rvC5NvQ8_

➤ Tips & key concepts

Parenchyma vs. Stroma

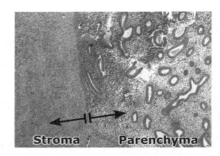

- **Parenchyma**: the functional cells of an organ (e.g., in kidney: renal tubules).
- **Stroma**: supportive framework of the organ (i.e., everything else, like connective tissue, blood vessels, etc.).
  - ○ Think: **Stroma** → "**straw-man**" (i.e., like straw, it's not functional – just structural).

Nuclei

Large nuclei generally mean more immature cells and faster cell division (which makes sense, as the nucleus contains DNA).

  - ○ Clinical correlate: This is highly clinically relevant because cancer cells, especially aggressive ones, generally have large nuclei and reproduce quickly.

Mature   Immature

Lipid Droplets

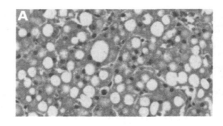

Empty, white balls generally represent **lipid droplets** 🅰. The lipid itself actually gets lost during routine preparation of histological slides, so the white blobs are areas devoid of stain, where the lipid used to be. Simply think of what oil droplets look like in water.

Types of Collagen

1. Type 1: Bone
   - ○ Think: any long bone looks like the number '1'. Alternative: *bONE*

2. Type 2: Cartilage
   - ○ Think: you have **2** ears (made of cartilage). Alternative: *Car2lage*

3. Type 3: Blood vessels
   - ○ Think: *l3lood* vessels

4. Type 4: Basement membrane

o   <u>Think</u>: type *four* forms the *floor* of tissues

5. Type 5: **Placenta**
    o   <u>Think</u>: type 5 is in *last place*

Epidermis layers

Remember the top and bottom layers using the following cues, and then just memorize the three layers in between. They are *(superficial to deep)*:

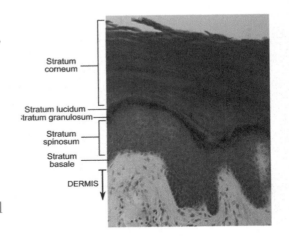

- **Stratum corneum:** think of the **cornea**, which is the *outermost* layer of the eye.
- Stratum lucidum
- Stratum granulosum
- Stratum spinosum
- **Stratum basale:** the name literally tells you it's the **basal** (bottom) layer.

Prussian blue stain

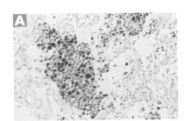

Prussian blue stains 🅰 show **iron** deposition (<u>think</u>: **Russians** like to pump **iron**).

Microtubule movements

- **Dynein:** retrograde
    o   <u>Think</u>: you don't want to **die** so you need to go back the other way (i.e., back away from death).
- **Kinesin:** anterograde
    o   Simply 'the other one'

NOTES

5. Ethics

Ethics in medical school teaches guidelines on how to approach and navigate certain tricky ethical scenarios as a physician.

Intensity: low

Memorization: 1/5

Content emphasis on board exams: medium-high

➤ Approach & guidelines

Studying other subjects concurrently

Ethics is perhaps the most understanding-heavy subject in medicine. This means it requires far less revision than memorization-heavy subjects. As such, a reasonable approach may be to sandwich it in between preparation for memorization-heavy subjects, allowing time for spaced repetition of those subjects.

For example, suppose you have both an anatomy and an ethics exam in two weeks. You can spend the first week and a half learning anatomy, then learn all of your ethics material in a couple of days, and then spend your last couple of days reviewing your anatomy (and perhaps have a very quick glance at ethics).

Overall approach

A good overall approach to consider for learning ethics is:

1. Learn your lecture/course material.
2. Review *First Aid*'s *Ethics* section (under 'Public Health Sciences').
3. Complete the 100 cases in "*Kaplan Medical USMLE Medical Ethics: The 100 Cases You Are Most Likely to See on the Exam*", OR, watch a commercial video series such as *Boards and Beyond*.

Generally, not too much else is needed for ethics, and the above three steps should be sufficient to do quite well in the subject. *First Aid* summarizes the most important ethical principles, and the Kaplan 100 Cases book should allow you to be quite well-prepared for most of the ethics questions you face in exams. If you opt not to use this book, you can go through a commercial video series in its place and that should be fine. Any remaining ethics preparation for your board exams (including the USMLE Step 1, MCCQE 1, and PLEB) should be adequately taken care of by your main question bank (UWorld, Kaplan, etc.)

Envisioning the ideal physician

Just like with clinical skills, an important part of selecting the correct response in ethics questions is being able to envision an empathetic and responsible physician in that scenario. It therefore helps to have at least a portion of your ethics learning come from listening to a (good) lecturer speak. Many students read out the answer choices in their mind in the voice of their lecturer to help guide them to the correct answer. This is indeed beneficial, and while this alone will not get you the answer for more complex questions, it does a great job in getting you most of the easier questions and eliminating incorrect answer choices quickly. Therefore, consider having one of your learning methods for ethics be either attending your class lectures or listening to a commercial video series (e.g., Kaplan, Boards and Beyond).

➤ Top resources

As mentioned, two of your top resources will be *First Aid*'s *Ethics* section and the book *Kaplan Medical USMLE Medical Ethics: The 100 Cases You Are Most Likely to See on the Exam*.

Any of the major video series (Kaplan, Boards and Beyond, Lecturio, DIT, etc.) will be sufficient, though the ethics lectures of **Boards and Beyond** and **Kaplan** are particularly well-regarded.

➤ Useful YouTube videos & series

Series: Ethics [Dirty Medicine]

This is an excellent series of 16 videos on the behavioral sciences. In addition to his easy-to-follow explanations, he also runs through questions to demonstrate the concepts. Note: there are a couple of videos in this series that are not exactly "ethics", namely the videos on insurance and the 6 stages of behavioral change.

➢   https://www.youtube.com/playlist?list=PL5rTEahBdxV5szNYtMDCm7YuiG51WUnZV

Series: USMLE STEP 1: COMMUNICATION [Randy Neil, MD]

Two 17- and 25-minute videos breaking down questions just Dirty Medicine's Ethics series above, except focused on empathy and communication.

➢   https://www.youtube.com/playlist?list=PLuyQGqW98ZltufEAnlpUuwqsaJ7-GOHYA

Series: USMLE STEP 1: ETHICS [Randy Neil, MD]

Two 18- and 20-minute videos in which Dr. Randy Neil goes over ethics questions and provides great breakdowns of how to approach them.

➢   https://www.youtube.com/playlist?list=PLuyQGqW98ZluosdiCSW_zeV8KKrgLf8K7

Ethics Principles [Boards and Beyond]

Not on YouTube but rather the Boards and Beyond website. Nonetheless, this is an excellent and high-yield 11-minute video highlighting important tips for navigating questions about autonomy, beneficence, non-maleficence, and justice. Pay especially close attention to the points in red.

➤ https://www.boardsbeyond.com/ethics-principles

➤ **Tips & key concepts**

Getting a deeper understanding

In an exam question with an ethical scenario involving a patient encounter, if you ever see an answer choice along the lines of "enquire why the patient feels/thinks that way so that you can make a more educated decision", strongly consider *that* answer.

Key concepts that are stressed these days are making educated decisions, attending to the patient's feelings/thoughts, and not rushing to hasty judgement.

Otherwise, there are a few exceptions to this in which you need to respond very directly but respectfully. These scenarios are usually obvious and involve the patient or a relative asking for or doing something blatantly unethical or unreasonable, e.g., the patient trying to hit on you or relatives asking you to continue life support despite the patient being officially brain dead.

Refusal to being told a diagnosis

Patients are allowed to refuse being told their diagnosis, but first find out *why* they feel that way. Their refusal may be rooted in a misconception, for example, about prognosis or treatment options.

Refusal of treatment or making a harmful choice

If a patient is refusing treatment or choosing something that is harmful to them, the correct approach is (in this order):

1. Find out *WHY* they're choosing that.
2. Express that you have concern about of the consequences of that choice (in a caring, non-threatening way).
3. Respect their final decision and autonomy and let them know you'll be there for them whenever they may need you.

Decisions about patient care

For board exams, the following is the order in which decisions about the patient's care are made:

1. Patient's words *right now* (as long as they have decision-making capacity).
2. Advance directive (e.g., living will) or medical power of attorney.
3. Surrogate decision-maker (spouse generally has highest priority).

Suspected abuse

If you see a child with their parent and you suspect the child is being abused, the correct answer is to literally take the child out of the room (e.g., you say something like "I'm just going to see him/her in the other room for a moment") and call child protective services.

"Consult the ethics committee"

This is almost always the wrong choice. They're asking YOU the question because YOU should have the capacity to recognize the right thing to do in the scenario. Remember: they're asking the question because they're testing an important underlying principle that you should know.

Ethics vs. legal question

Read the question and try to determine whether it's a question focusing on ethics or law. If it's ethics, consider the most caring, least judgmental, and most responsible answer choice. If it's legal, go with the most straightforward, by-the-book answer, which usually is a fact or law you just have to memorize/know.

6. Epidemiology and Biostatistics

Epidemiology is the study of health and disease in *populations*, and biostatistics is about research methods in medicine. They guide the practice of medicine by allowing us to determine what treatments work better than others, amongst other things. For this reason, they'll be very important to you regardless of what specialty you pursue. Many residency programs actually require residents to complete a research project during their residency and, as a physician, you'll need to know how to interpret research studies and draw conclusions from them.

Intensity: low-medium

Memorization: 3/5

Content emphasis on board exams: high

> **➤ Approach & guidelines**

Compared to most basic science subjects, there isn't a lot of content in epidemiology and biostatistics. But it is *very* high-yield for both board exams and real-life clinical research. This makes the subject very high-reward relative to the time investment required.

The bulk of the important content of epidemiology and biostatistics is contained within First Aid's *Public Health Sciences* chapter. If you genuinely understand this information and know how to apply it, you will have a reasonably good understanding for the basic sciences level, and you'll be prepared for most board exam questions. Therefore, consider an approach along these lines:

1. Have a quick skim through *First Aid's Epidemiology & Biostatistics* section.
2. Learn the material well from your course **lectures** OR a commercial **video series** and follow along in your *First Aid*.

   o Annotate with any new important information you learn
   o Supplement your learning with YouTube videos

3. Complete **practice questions** from a major question bank (e.g., Kaplan, UWorld).

If you've already completed your epidemiology and biostatistics course and just want to do a thorough review of the subject, consider completing a commercial video series like Kaplan or Boards and Beyond at 1.5x-1.75x speed. Alternatively, if you learned the subject very well the first time around, you could simply go through your annotated *First Aid*.

Equations

Review epidemiology equations in the moments before the exam. Once you take your seat at the testing center, write down all equations on the sheet of paper they provide you. Then, in the heat of the test, if your mind becomes clouded or you're short on time, you'll have them in writing to quickly refer to. It may also be useful to write down the percentages for 1, 2, and 3 standard deviations (68%, 95%, 99.7%, respectively) and the Z scores for the 95% and 99% confidence intervals (1.96 and 2.58, respectively), as these can be easy to confuse.

➤ Top resources

Aside from *First Aid*, you don't particularly need many additional resources for epidemiology and biostatistics. YouTube videos can help polish your understanding and make various concepts easier to wrap your head around, and commercial video series can help you do a good top-to-bottom review if needed. The epidemiology and biostatistics video lectures of **Kaplan** and **Boards and Beyond** are particularly well-regarded, but you should be fine with any of the major companies.

➤ Useful YouTube channels

Rahul Patwari

Rahul Patwari is an excellent lecturer who has videos on both clinical medicine and epidemiology/biostatistics. His videos cover high-yield concepts (see *Useful YouTube videos and series* below), but some videos may also delve into more supplementary information.

➤ https://www.youtube.com/user/oldblueday

Randy Neil, MD

Randy Neil runs through high-yield USMLE-style questions and explains the reasoning behind the answer choices really well. Listed in *Useful YouTube videos and series* are some of his best epidemiology videos, however he has more aside from these on his channel in case you wanted to explore.

➤ https://www.youtube.com/channel/UCjTHgZY7U6pajEz61sQCHBw

Series: USMLE BIOSTATS QUICK REVIEW Q's [Randy Neil, MD]

> https://www.youtube.com/playlist?list=PLuyQGqW98ZlvLuI6muv8T7ue6EnD11CyS

Attack Rates and Case-Fatality Rates [Rahul Patwari]

> https://www.youtube.com/watch?v=2_qKgbLOlyY

Clinical Reasoning 09: Sensitivity, Specificity, and Predictive Values [Rahul Patwari]

Thorough and intuitive explanation of sensitivity, specificity, and positive and negative predictive values.

> https://www.youtube.com/watch?v=pUa08fB_AN4

Incidence and prevalence [Rahul Patwari]

> https://www.youtube.com/watch?v=Xd01PXsUdBc&t=19s

Odds Ratio and Risk Ratio [Rahul Patwari]

> https://www.youtube.com/watch?v=hOtoV2Kjb0o

Screening tests [Rahul Patwari]

> https://www.youtube.com/watch?v=VZjxmrB2S8I

The Relationship Between Incidence and Prevalence [Rahul Patwari]

> https://www.youtube.com/watch?v=1jzZe3ORdd8

Biostatistics SUMMARY Step 1 – The Basics USMLE [Randy Neil, MD]

A really helpful video in which Dr. Neil goes through several high-yield statistics questions and gives brilliant walk-throughs for each. Highly recommended!

> https://www.youtube.com/watch?v=75pQPB1RF50

Biostatistics SUMMARY Step 1 – USMLE The Extra stuff [Randy Neil, MD]

Part 2 of the previous video. This is not quite as high-yield as part 1, but is still useful.

> https://www.youtube.com/watch?v=VMI9UuNqoGI

USMLE STEP 1: BIAS & CONFOUNDING w/ QUESTIONS [Randy Neil, MD]

Another video by Dr. Neil running through questions dealing with the different biases.

> https://www.youtube.com/watch?v=wt1Xy9y1bXM

> **Tips & key concepts**

Sensitivity vs. specificity

Possibly the single most important concept of epidemiology and biostatistics is the idea of the **sensitivity** and **specificity** of a test. You must understand these two terms thoroughly and ensure you don't mix them up. This is not hard if you simply think about the *meaning of each word*:

Sensitivity

Think of a *sensitive alarm system*. An alarm that is very sensitive is one that is very easily set off. The benefit of this is that you're very like to catch the "bad guy" (or in medicine, any disease). Screening tests need to be sensitive, so you don't miss anything.

Specificity

An alarm is specific if it is only set off by a bad guy and not, for example, by a passing animal, the rain or by a gust of wind. It *specifically* singles out bad guys. In a medical test, this means the test is specific to that one disease only, i.e., if the test comes back positive, you can be pretty certain it's not due to some other disease or trigger.

Confirmatory tests must be specific because you want to confirm that previous positive tests were not caused by other things, and that the patient really does have that specific disease.

There often isn't a single test that's both highly sensitive and specific. Sometimes you have an amazingly sensitive test with trash specificity, or vice versa. For this reason, disease detection is often done in 2 stages: screening tests and confirmatory tests. You start with a highly sensitive screening test and catch the vast majority of disease cases but also a few who do not really have the disease (false positives). You then do highly specific confirmatory testing to get rid of any of those false positives.

Sensitivity/specificity vs. negative/positive predictive values

Sensitivity and specificity are intrinsic properties of a test and do <u>*not*</u> change with disease prevalence. Think of the previous alarm system example – how sensitive or specific an alarm is doesn't change and is just a matter of how the alarm was made.

Positive and negative predictive values, however, DO change with disease prevalence because as their names imply, they involve making <u>*predictions*</u> about the results in a given population. For example, if the test predicts that someone has a disease in a population where 99% of all people have that disease, that prediction is most likely correct (i.e., high positive predictive value)!

On the other hand, if a test predicts someone to have a disease in a population where its prevalence is one in a million, you might seriously question that prediction (i.e., low positive predictive value). In other words, it might be more likely that the positive result was just a mistake of the test rather than the patient actually having that super uncommon disease.

Cohort vs. case-control study: *think of the names*

- **Cohort study:** starts with a **cohort** (a group of people with shared characteristics i.e., exposures or risk factors) and sees how many go/went on to develop the disease (**past →future**).
- **Case-control study:** the name literally tells you it starts with **cases** (patients with disease), and then checks to see how many were exposed to a given risk factor in the past (**future → past**).

Relative risk vs. odds ratio

An *extremely* commonly tested concept that you WILL see many questions on is the measures of likelihood for cohort vs. case-control studies. They are:

1. **Cohort:** relative risk (RR)
2. **Case-control:** odds ratio (OR)

You can remember this by simply thinking of the word *"risk"*. Patients in case-control studies *already have the disease* – you can't assess the risk of something you already have! You *can*, however, assess the risk of developing a disease later (= cohort study).

NOTES

7. Biochemistry

Biochemistry in medical school is centered on the biochemical pathways related to diseases. It's one of the most hated subjects in medical school, so don't feel too bad if you don't enjoy studying it. You likely won't encounter fine biochemistry details much in clinical practice for most specialties. It is important for lab-based medical research though, if you have an interest in that.

<u>Intensity</u>: medium-high

<u>Memorization</u>: 4.5/5

<u>Content emphasis on board exams</u>: low-medium

> **Approach & guidelines**

Since a good chunk of biochemistry is usually seen by students in their undergraduate years, it may be tempting to study the course the way you did in undergrad, or to even use the same textbooks or notes that worked for you back then. This would be an enormous mistake. While many of the topics you learn might be similar (e.g., glycolysis, Krebs, amino acids, etc.), both the level of detail and the content emphasis are entirely different.

Biochemistry in medical school is generally briefer and is highly clinically oriented. You simply don't have time to waste on all the little clinically irrelevant details they teach you in undergrad. It is therefore important to let most of those former approaches, textbooks, and notes go, as counterintuitive as it might seem.

Consider the following general strategy:

1. Have a quick skim through *First Aid's Biochemistry* section and this chapter's *Tips and Key Concepts* section (see page 115).
2. Learn the material well from your course **lectures** OR a commercial **video series** and follow along in your *First Aid*.

   o Annotate with any new important information you learn.
   o Revisit this chapter's *Tips and Key Concepts* section when you encounter a topic that's mentioned therein.

   o Supplement your learning with YouTube videos.

3. Complete **practice questions** (e.g., BRS, Kaplan, UWorld).

First Aid's biochemistry section is quite long and thorough, and by annotating it with any additional high-yield information, it can be sufficient for board exam preparation. You generally don't have to buy an additional review book for biochemistry unless you genuinely want to (see *Top Resources* below for options). Avoid over-annotating and flooding your *First Aid* with low-yield information (of which there can be a ton of in biochemistry!). When you return to it to review the subject, you want your review process to be pleasant and efficient – not long and burdensome.

Pay ***especially*** close attention to concepts related to diseases. The following are very high-yield topics:

- Carbohydrate metabolism disorders (fructose, galactose, lactose, sorbitol).
- Glycogen storage diseases.
- Lysosomal storage diseases.
- Ketone bodies (very important, as it's related to diabetes!). You MUST know
  - the two main ketone bodies – B-hydroxybutyrate and acetoacetate;
  - that in diabetic ketoacidosis and starvation, there is an *increase in the B-hydroxybutyrate:acetoacetate ratio.*
  - that urine ketone tests detect *acetoacetate* but not B-hydroxybutyrate (<u>think</u>: <u>u</u>*rine and* <u>a</u>*cetoacetate both start with vowels*).
- Lipoprotein functions (e.g., LDL, VLDL).
- The catecholamine synthesis pathway and amino acid-related disorders (e.g., alkaptonuria, phenylketonuria, etc.).
- The homocysteine pathway and the involvement of vitamins B6 and B12 in it.
- Hexokinase vs. glucokinase.
- All vitamin and mineral deficiencies.

Connecting pathways

First Aid has an excellent "Summary of Pathways" page in their *Biochemistry* section that shows all of the major pathways and the relationships between each. This page is invaluable in helping you get a firm understanding of where each pathway stands in the "big picture" of things, and what the highest-yield enzymes and cofactors are within them. Therefore, refer back to this page throughout your learning of the various individual pathways.

Question banks

Completing quality practice questions is particularly important for biochemistry because of how easy it is to get caught up in the plethora of details and lose sight of the critical take-away points.

You have two primary choices: *BRS Biochemistry, Molecular Biology, and Genetics'* end-of-chapter quizzes or a USMLE question bank such as Kaplan or UWorld. Given that the *BRS* end-of-chapter quizzes are shorter in length, they can be particularly useful for ensuring you've solidified the most important facts and concepts for each major topic in rapid-fire fashion. As such, they may be better suited to helping you pass and excel in your school's biochemistry course. Biochemistry questions from a USMLE question bank, on the other hand, contain more depth and are better for preparing for major board exams and for reinforcing the most clinically important facts and concepts.

> **Top resources**

As usual, two of your top resources will be **First Aid** and **YouTube**. Depending on the quality of your school's lectures, you may or may not want to use a video course to learn the subject.

Some students also like **Dr. Najeeb** lectures, especially because they're free and available on YouTube. However, his videos are often _very_ long, and for a subject that is not too high-yield like biochemistry, it is most likely *NOT* worth your time. Other video series can usually cover the same content in significantly less time. Nonetheless, consider a video of his if you're really struggling with a particular concept and need a clear explanation.

Review books

Some students may also opt to get a review book for biochemistry. As mentioned previously, this is entirely optional (and especially if you're using a video course, it's most likely overkill), as *First Aid's* biochemistry section is quite long and thorough. If you do want to consider one though, your top choices are:

BRS Biochemistry, Molecular Biology, and Genetics (Lieberman and Ricer)

The BRS book series is well-liked by many students and is up to date (7th edition from 2019). 448 pages. Contains excellent questions at the end of each chapter.

Rapid Review Biochemistry (Pelley and Goljan)

One of the shortest biochemistry review books (~200 pages). Well organized. The downside is that it's fairly old (2010).

Again, these review books are **_not necessary_** to learn biochemistry, so if you're considering them, scan through a library copy or use Amazon's *Look Inside* feature to see if you feel they would truly benefit you.

Other

Pixorize (www.pixorize.com)

An additional resource that can be helpful in memorizing some particularly hard facts or pathways is **Pixorize** videos. Pixorize makes visual mnemonics in the form of scenes with stories (similar to Sketchy Medical). Since these types of mnemonics work best for memorization-heavy subjects, they can be effective for some areas of biochemistry. It might be wise not to over-rely on Pixorize though, as their sketches can be hit or miss. Consider them on a sketch-to-sketch basis. Many of their sketches are on YouTube (see *Useful YouTube channels*).

➤ Useful YouTube channels

Dirty Medicine

Dirty Medicine has numerous videos on biochemistry in which he explains important concepts in easy-to-follow ways, with emphasis on content that's high-yield for the USMLE step 1.

➤ https://www.youtube.com/channel/UCZaDAUF7UEcRXIFvGZu3O9Q

Pixorize

As discussed above, Pixorize makes visual mnemonics in the form of sketches with stories. They have some videos for biochemistry.

➤ https://www.youtube.com/channel/UCpciEfaGm95mWt5L2jRi6ww

➤ Useful YouTube videos & series

Series: Biochemistry & Genetics [Dirty Medicine]

A series of 30 easy-to-follow videos on the major processes and concepts in biochemistry (along with a few genetics videos thrown in).

➤ https://www.youtube.com/playlist?list=PL5rTEahBdxV6prB_iWNU8N2-L5XAktld8

Series: Biochemistry | Medical Education Video [Lecturio]

A video series by Lecturio on biochemistry. This series does not have everything (its focus seems to be amino acids and enzymes). If you're already going through a video course like Kaplan or Boards and Beyond, it would probably be wise to just stick with that course.

➤ https://www.youtube.com/playlist?list=PLVnjTkEwv-uMN7iB8phOMLDV7TS9luqtK

Series: Pixorize Biochemistry [Pixorize]

Pixorize's USMLE videos on biochemistry.

➤ https://www.youtube.com/playlist?list=PLtVla_HPRH_t5PM-J50fGlzZy_9AOnrJ7

Series: USMLE Biochemistry [Randy Neil, MD]

A series of 7 videos by Dr. Neil in which he works through problems centered on the catecholamine/tyrosine pathway (a very high-yield pathway). You may not need to watch all of them but watching a couple can be really helpful to solidify your understanding of the pathway and develop the right thought process.

➤ https://www.youtube.com/playlist?list=PLuyQGqW98Zlvlv77QEtB1WPGzbR14msNE

Hexokinase vs. glucokinase

- **Hexokinase**: Sequesters glucose in the tissue for use. Present in **most tissues**. Predominant at *low* glucose concentrations.
  - Think: **H**exokinase ➔ **E**xercise (used in more than just exercise, but this should remind you that hexokinase predominates when your tissues are in need of glucose for energy)
- **Glucokinase**: Starts the process of glycogen synthesis by storing excess glucose in the liver when glucose concentrations are *high*. Present only in **liver** and **β cells of pancreas**.
  - Think: **Glu**cokinase ➔ **Glu**es glucose together to form glycogen

Kinases

- For all three major monosaccharide metabolism pathways (glucose, galactose, and fructose), the first enzyme is a "*-kinase*" (glucokinase/hexokinase, galactokinase, fructokinase, respectively). This is because kinases **trap sugar inside the cell** by phosphorylating it.
- For disorders of both fructose and galactose metabolism, the milder condition is when the defect is in the "kinase" enzyme.
  - This makes sense as the kinase enzymes carry out the first step of each pathway. If you can't start that pathway, it's not that big of a deal – you're pretty much just left with the sugar, which you can pee out.
  - On the other hand, defects in enzymes further down the line mean you have a problem *after* you've already committed to the pathway – you've spent energy and you've **trapped the sugar inside the cell** through phosphorylation. This is much worse…
  - Think: disorders of the **kin**ase enzymes are much **kin**der.

Energy sources

- Red blood cells use *only glycolysis* (no oxygen/oxidative phosphorylation) for energy because they have no mitochondria.
  - Think: their job is to *CARRY* oxygen, so you don't want them to *USE* the oxygen.
- The brain only uses glucose and ketone bodies for energy – *not fat*. This is because fatty acid-albumin complexes are very large and cannot cross the blood-brain barrier.

Sorbitol

Sorbitol causes **osmotic** damage to tissues (it causes cells to ab**sorb** too much water).

Nutritional deficiencies (highest yield associations)

Nutrient	Deficiency pathology	Mnemonic
Vitamin A	**Eye** and **skin** problems (especially remember night blindness, Bitot spots, corneal degeneration, and dry skin)	*'A'* being the *first letter* of the alphabet, think about the *first* (outer-most) *parts of your body*: eyes and skin
Vitamin D	**Bone** problems (children → rickets **A**; adults → osteomalacia)	*"D for Deformity"*, or simply remember vitamin D's association with calcium metabolism
Vitamin E	**Hemolytic anemia** and **neurologic problems** (B12 deficiency mimic)	*"E for Entioxidant"*. Without antioxidants, two of your most important cells – RBCs and neurons – get destroyed by free radicals
Vitamin K	**Bleeding**	"**K** for **K**oagulation"
Vitamin B₁	**Nervous tissue damage** (brain in Wernicke-Korsakoff syndrome [usually alcohol-related], peripheral neurons in dry beriberi)	**B1→** point to your brain with **1** finger (i.e., making the "think!" sign) to remember brain and nerve damage. Additionally, spell beriberi as "*Ber1Ber1*" (**B1**)
		Don't forget *wet beriberi*, which causes dilated cardiomyopathy (you can point to your heart with *1* finger, making the "it comes from the heart" motion).
Vitamin B₃	**Pellagra**	**B3→ 3** D's (**D**iarrhea, **D**ementia, **D**ermatitis)
Vitamin B₆	**Peripheral neuropathy**	**B6** → grab your thumb with your opposite hand (= **6** fingers in total) like you just hurt it to remember peripheral neuropathy (presents as pain/numbness in hands/feet)
Vitamin B₉ (folate)	**Neural tube defects** in pregnancy	Lack of **folate** will **foil** your pregnancy
Vitamin B₁₂	**Subacute combined degeneration** (spinal cord degeneration)	If you had to wake up at **midnight** (*12* i.e., B12), you'd be all **weak** and **off-balance** (→ reminds you of dorsal column, corticospinal tract, and spinocerebellar tract involvement)
		Remember: **S**ubacute **C**ombined **D**egeneration → **S**pinocerebellar tracts, **C**orticospinal tracts, and **D**orsal columns degenerate
Both vitamin B₉ and B₁₂	**Megaloblastic anemia**	The two vitamins with the **biggest** numbers (9 and 12) cause **big RBCs**
Protein	**Kwashiorkor:** peripheral and abdominal edema	Kwashiorkor makes you **edematous** and gives you a swollen belly (ascites) as low blood albumin causes low oncotic pressure and fluid leakage into abdominal cavity, while marasmus – energy deficiency – does NOT
		Think: **Kwashi**-orkor → **squashy** belly

Catecholamine synthesis enzymes and diseases

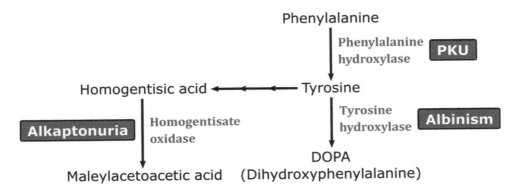

- **Phenyl**ketonuria: **phenyl**alanine hydroxylase deficiency
  - Think: in **phenyl**ketonuria, you smell, look, and think **phunny** [*funny*] (= musty body odor, growth retardation/microcephaly, intellectual disability).
- **Alkap**tonuria: homo**gent**isate oxidase deficiency
  - Think: **Al Kapone** was a real **gent**leman (probably not though.....!)
    - Bonus: remember alkaptonuria causes bluish-black connective tissue by picturing Al Capone being bluish black from all the gunpowder residue and soot of firing his gun so much(!)
- **Albinism**: tyrosine hydroxylase deficiency
  - Think: The *"tyre"* in **tyr**osine should remind you that it's dealing with pigment (every tire is black – have you ever in your life seen one that isn't?) Therefore, a defect in tyrosine hydroxylase will obviously cause a defect in pigmenting the skin.

Electron transport chain complex inhibitors

- **Complex 1**: rotenone
- **Complex 3**: antimycin A
  - Think: the **antichrist** is a prominent concept in **Trinitarian** ("**3**") Christianity.
- **Complex 4**: cyanide, CO
  - Think: complex **4** inhibitors → poisons commonly used by people who think they have nothing else to live **4**.
- **Complex 5**: oligomycin
  - Think: **oligomycin** sounds like "**only a little more to go**" (i.e., it inhibits the *last* complex).

Lysosomal storage diseases – enzyme mnemonics

- **Tay-Sachs disease:** He**X**osaminidase A
  - Think: Spell it Tay-Sa**X**.
- **Fabry disease:** α-galactosidase A

- o   Think: A kid named **Fabry** who's totally wimpy and not **alpha.**
- **Metachromatic leukodystrophy:** aryl**sulf**atase A
  - o   Think: **Sulfur** is a **colorful** substance (it's yellow) (*chromatic* means 'relating to *color*').
- **Krabbe disease:** galacto**cerebrosidase**
  - o   Think: A **crab**-shaped **galaxy.**
- **Niemann-Pick disease:** sphingomyelinase
  - o   Think: who **picked** the **name** for the **Sphinx**? It really is a hard name to pronounce… (alternatively, picture the **Sphinx** being carved out with a **pick**axe).
- **Hunter vs. Hurler syndrome:** iduronate sulfatase and α–L-iduronidase, respectively
  - o   Think: Both have "iduron-" in the name, so just remember: you have to **hunt** (i.e., go mining) for **sulfur** (**sulfa**tase). Think of Hurler syndrome as 'the other one' or remember α–L-iduronidase is for the one with an 'L' in the name (hur**L**er).

8. Genetics

Genetics in medical school teaches you principles of disease inheritance, common genetic conditions and chromosomal abnormalities, lab techniques, and some random genetics facts about diseases (e.g., disease's chromosomal association). Some of it is important for any physician to know – namely, principles of inheritance, Down syndrome, and a *rough* understanding of lab techniques. Some of it is mostly only applicable to geneticists and researchers in certain specialties (e.g., diseases' chromosomal associations).

Intensity: low

Memorization: 4/5

Using pedigrees to determine modes of inheritance is understanding-heavy; almost everything else in genetics is memorization-heavy.

Content emphasis on board exams: low-medium

> ➤ **Approach & guidelines**

Genetics – at least at medical school level – is a relatively simple subject, but there are two main areas some students struggle with:

1. Solving pedigree problems, and
2. Memorizing genetic facts for diseases (e.g., chromosome numbers, modes of transmission).

Solving pedigree problems

Exceling in pedigree problems is not just a matter of being able to figure out the solution – it's about figuring it out *quickly*. To do so, you need a simple system to approach every problem with (see below), and you need to do a decent number of practice questions to learn to apply the system quickly.

There are several common pitfalls and misconceptions with pedigree problems, and it takes practice to avoid making them.

Use this 3-step strategy to quickly solve pedigrees:

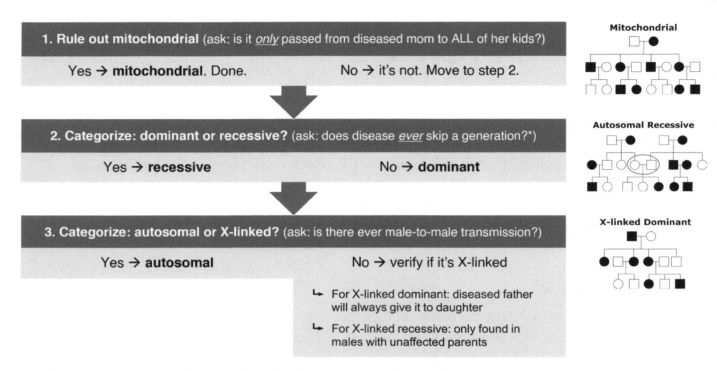

*Another way to ask question 2 is: "Does any diseased patient have two normal parents?"

Memorizing genetic facts

There are two frustrating aspects that must be memorized: **chromosome number** and **mode of transmission**.

Chromosome numbers

You have two options in memorizing chromosome numbers: brute repetition or number mnemonics (see *5. Mnemonics* on page 46). You may not be able to think of a good number mnemonic for every disorder, but they can be effective when you do. For example, to remember Friedreich ataxia occurring on chromosome 9, you can picture a cat (*represents 9 ["9 lives"]*) eating fried rice (*Friedreich*). Another example: to remember hemochromatosis occurring on chromosome 6, you can picture a dice (*represents 6*) made of iron (*hemochromatosis*) or that's rusted.

Modes of transmission

It's generally more effective to memorize the mode of disease transmission when you're learning the actual disease rather than just trying to memorize a large list of, for example, autosomal dominant disorders. Therefore, unless you will be tested on this information in your school's genetics course, leave it for when you encounter that disease in its respective organ system (e.g., memorize hemophilia A and B being X-linked recessive when you study it in hematology).

A useful method for memorizing modes of transmission is to create a recurring symbol for each mode and visualize the disease somehow relating to it. For example, you might choose to represent 'autosomal recessive' by visualizing a shy or hiding patient. Then, you can picture an albino man being shy of his condition or hiding from the sun, or a child with sickle cell disease hiding from a sickle-wielding maniac. It can take practice to become good at doing this, but it can be very effective! But, if you're pressed for time, consider memorizing using just brute repetition, as modes of transmission are usually not too high-yield anyways.

A useful supplement you can consider for memorizing both modes of transmission of genetic diseases and their chromosome numbers (if relevant) is Sketchy Medical's pathology videos. They often incorporate a visual mnemonic for both of these. This is entirely a matter of convenience, though, and is much more feasible if you either already have a subscription or plan to get one soon for pathology. Don't spend money on an entire Sketchy subscription just for genetics.

Genetic disorders

When learning genetic disorders, consider a YouTube search for real patients with the disorder. Seeing a real patient can work wonders to help you understand and remember the disorder in ways a book or PowerPoint slide can't.

Learn the trisomy syndromes well, as these are high-yield. In particular, KNOW EVERYTHING about **Down syndrome** and take your sweet time learning it, as it is *extremely* high-yield for board exams. You need to know the three main ways in which Down syndrome occurs (meiotic nondisjunction, unbalanced Robertsonian translocation, and mosaicism) and that **meiotic nondisjunction** is by far the most common of the three. Also have a rough understanding how each of these three processes work. In addition to the trisomy syndromes, **cystic fibrosis** is another favorite topic for board exam questions, so be sure to learn it well.

Genetics terms

To remember all of the various genetics terms (heteroplasmy, locus heterogeneity, etc.), spend time reflecting on each of their names. In most cases, the name will tell you exactly what the term means and will save you from having to blindly memorize. For example, "**uniparental disomy**" tells you **one parent** (*uniparental*) gives **2** (*di-*) copies of a chromo**some** (*-somy*).

Lab techniques

If your school teaches lab techniques, such as PCR, blotting procedures, etc., as part of their genetics course, invest time into developing a decent general understanding of them, because they'll keep reappearing throughout your basic sciences. Do NOT waste your time on the fine procedural details – much more important is to have a *general* image in your mind of how each test works.

Pay particular attention to **polymerase chain reaction** (PCR), **enzyme-linked immunosorbent assay** (ELISA), and **flow cytometry,** as these often come up in exams and in clinical medicine.

Be sure to learn the "SNoW DRoP" mnemonic for blotting procedures, as this will score you a lot of points in the long run:

SNoW DRoP
Southern = DNA
Northern = RNA
Western = Protein

➤ Top resources

Given how brief genetics is in medical school, it's probably not worth buying a textbook. *First Aid* contains most of the genetics you need to know, and supplementing that with YouTube videos, a commercial video series, or your school lectures is usually more than enough.

As discussed previously, **Sketchy Pathology** videos can help you memorize the mode of transmission and/or chromosome number of a genetic disease. If you already have a subscription or plan to get one soon for your pathology course, consider using it. However, it's definitely not worth buying a subscription solely for genetics.

➤ Useful YouTube channels

Osmosis

Osmosis has videos on various genetic diseases that can serve as very good starting points when learning them, as their explanations are very clear and visually appealing. These include Down syndrome, Cri du chat syndrome, primary mitochondrial myopathy, Freidreich ataxia, and more. Keep in mind some videos go into a bit more detail than necessary for medical school (e.g., discussing complex molecular genetics), so use what you need from their videos and simply skip over the extra parts.

➤ https://www.youtube.com/osmosis/

➤ Useful YouTube videos & series

Bintang crying (Cri du chat syndrome) [Bintang Yasa]

A super memorable video of a real patient with Cri du chat syndrome that will stick with you for a long time.

➤ https://www.youtube.com/watch?v=0K78eRSqDkk

Hardy-Weinberg Equation [Bozeman Science]

A very good explanation of how to use the Hardy-Weinberg equation, in case you needed to polish up on this concept.

➤ https://www.youtube.com/watch?v=oEBNom3K9cQ

Prader-Willi vs. Angelman Syndrome (Imprinting) [Dirty Medicine]

A concise explanation of the highest-yield points of the two imprinting syndromes.

➤ https://www.youtube.com/watch?v=VYbL_CQx2Dk

Genetics Terms [Dirty Medicine]

A concise run-through and explanation of the major genetics terms in 13 minutes.

➤ https://www.youtube.com/watch?v=xA3-pIUUQWg

Down syndrome (trisomy 21) – causes, symptoms, diagnosis, & pathology [Osmosis]

A brilliant explanation of the 3 modes of acquiring Down syndrome (nondisjunction, Robertsonian translocation, mosaicism).

➤ https://www.youtube.com/watch?v=ze_6VWwLtOE

➤ **Tips & key concepts**

Trisomy syndromes

The 3 trisomy syndromes are in reverse alphabetical order (Down syndrome has the highest number [21], Patau has the lowest [13]). I personally remembered **Edward** syndrome being trisomy **18** by thinking of **Squidward** (sounds like Edward) from Spongebob, who despite his name is actually an **octo**pus.

Trisomy 16 is the most common cause of chromosomal cause of miscarriage.

Nucleotide repeat expansion diseases

Memorize the four trinucleotide repeat expansion diseases well, as these can score you easy points on exams. Use this set of mnemonics:

- **Hunt**ington: "**C**an't **A**im **G**reat" (**CAG**)
  - o Picture a **hunt**er not being able to aim his gun well because of his chorea
- Myotonic dystrophy: "**C**hronic **T**onic **G**rip" (**CTG**)
  - o Myotonia is an impairment in muscle relaxation
- Fragile X syndrome: "**C**hin, **G**iant **G**onads" (**CGG**)
  - o Fragile X patients have large jaws and testes
- Friedreich ataxia: "**G**ait **A**lways **A**wkward" (**GAA**)
  - o Friedreich *ataxia* patients have *ataxic* gaits

Mitochondrial inheritance

Remember that mitochondrial inheritance is from mother to kids (you can also think: "mi-to-chondrial → mother-to-kids [or children]").

9. Microbiology

Medical microbiology is the study of microscopic organisms – namely, bacteria, viruses, fungi, and parasites – and how they cause disease.

Like anatomy, microbiology is another foundational subject that will carry over well to almost any specialty you choose. This is because almost every specialty deals with infectious disease in some scope, whether it's in the form of its treatment, prevention, management of its complications, or simply knowing how a given pathogen interacts with your organ system of specialty.

<u>Intensity</u>: high

<u>Memorization</u>: 5/5

<u>Content emphasis on board exams</u>: high

➤ Approach & guidelines

As with all your courses, your immediate priority is to pass the course. Therefore, there's no way around learning your course's lecture material. For microbiology, however, you *WILL* need supplementary resources to do well given how much non-intuitive information there is to be memorized and mentally organized. Unless you have an excellent professor and great lecture slides, consider learning the content from your supplementary resources *first*, and then return to your slides to pick up any missing pieces and prepare for your school exam.

Learning microbiology can be divided into two parts: **learning general principles** and **memorizing organisms**. Learning general principles should obviously come *first*, as it will assist you in memorizing organisms.

1. Learning general principles

Learning the general principles of microbiology (e.g., bacterial/viral structures and genetics) can be accomplished through a mix of your course lectures and slides, *First Aid*, YouTube videos, and/or a commercial video series (*if* you already have a subscription – *don't buy one just for this*). You definitely don't need *all* of these resources – find the couple that work best for you.

The extent to which you rely on your course lectures depends on their quality. If they're excellent in helping you understand the material, learn from them as a primary source. If not, learn the content from other sources and then return to your course's lecture slides to ensure you're prepared for your school exams.

Pay especially close attention to bacterial and viral genetics, as well as hepatitis serologic interpretation, as these are board exam favorites. The latter is also highly clinically relevant.

2. Memorizing organisms

For memorizing organisms, the approach is very simple: **Sketchy Medical**. Sketchy Medical makes sketches with narrations that help you remember information using visual cues. It's exceptionally effective for microbiology given the amount of pure memorization required in the subject. Their microbiology series (their original series) also happens to be one of their best. It makes learning microbiology quite fun, which is a significant advantage in the long run of your course given the enormous amount of study time it requires.

How to use *Sketchy*

Sketchy will be immensely helpful in the short term (e.g., up until your block exam) regardless of the specific approach you use with it. However, using it *strategically* is critical to your long-term retention and success in microbiology.

Timing

Firstly, use spaced repetition. This is especially important with Sketchy because it's centered on visual mnemonics and symbolism. You need to not only remember what symbols are in the sketch, but to also reinforce their meanings. This takes significant time and repetition, but once you do, it will pay off enormously. Microbiology will then be one of your strongest subjects and will require much less dedicated review time for major board exams. For this reason, it's important to start watching the relevant Sketchy videos *early* in your block exam preparation.

For example, suppose you have a block exam every 3 weeks in your microbiology course. A reasonable approach may look something like this:

1. Make it a goal to watch all the relevant Sketchy videos for that block exam (e.g., all viruses) in the first week, and make notes.
2. Review each sketch the day after you watch it. Try to recall each symbol and decipher its meaning *first* before checking your annotations.
3. Review all pertinent sketches a day or two before the block exam.
4. Review all sketches within a week of the final exam.

Annotation

To easily refer to Sketchy in the future, you may want to have each sketch and its meanings compiled in picture and written form. This way, you can refer to the information you need quickly without having to skim through an entire video. You have two main options for this: making an **electronic compilation** yourself or buying the *Sketchy Micro* **workbook**.

Electronic copy

The main advantage of making an electronic copy is the speed at which you can search for and find the information you need (done with a simple Ctrl + F search). The downside is that it takes *a lot* of time to make. To make an electronic copy:

1. Open a Sketchy video
2. Take a screenshot of the completed sketch (end of the video)
3. Paste the screenshot in a PowerPoint slide (trim the image as needed)
4. Duplicate the slide and annotate this second one.

This leaves you with a single file that you can easily search or go through and test yourself with. The reason for making two slides for each sketch – one blank and one annotated – is to be able to test yourself using the blank slide and decipher what each symbol means on your own before revealing the annotation.

Consider adding your own image mnemonics to the slides to remember any information that isn't mentioned. For example, Epstein-Barr Virus (infectious mono) classically causes T cells to look like ballerina skirts, so you can insert a ballerina skirt into the sketch.

Importantly though, when adding your own images, try to use images with transparent backgrounds where possible. Go to Google Images and click *'Tools'* – then click *'Color'* and select *'Transparent'*. This will show you images that contain just the object and no background. This way, when you copy and paste the picture into the slide, you get only the object (e.g., a potato) and not a rectangle picture (e.g., a picture of a potato on a table), making it look far better and less out-of-place. The more it blends in with the sketch, the better it works. For the same reason, see if you can find cartoon images of the object first – if not, real images can work.

Note: if you choose this option, I don't encourage sharing the file with others. The SketchyMedical team work hard for their money and make amazing products, so please do bear their rights in mind.

Sketchy Micro workbook

The *Sketchy Micro* workbook, bought from the Sketchy website, is simply a book with all of the sketches printed out and with space to annotate it. The downside is this book *DOES NOT* contain the annotations - you have to write them out yourself.

Question banks

When first learning microbiology, you will have your hands full. You may not have much time to go through a lot of questions, and that is entirely okay. As mentioned before, Sketchy Micro is an investment that will benefit you massively in the long term, but it does take a lot of time to run through and memorize initially.

With whatever time you do have to spare before your block exam, try to run through either the end-of-chapter quizzes in the **BRS Microbiology and Immunology** textbook or some USMLE question bank (e.g., UWorld, Kaplan) questions. *BRS* questions would generally be preferred when first learning microbiology as they're much shorter and you can run through them in rapid-fire fashion.

Highest-yield organisms

Some pathogens are extremely high-yield for both board exams and real-life medicine, either because of how common, dangerous, or versatile they are. Spend extra time on these pathogens and make sure you learn and remember them well, as they will come up again and again all throughout your studies. These include:

Bacteria

- *Staphylococcus aureus*
  - *S. aureus* can do almost anything; it's the most common cause of hospital-acquired infections and has developed major antibiotic resistance (MRSA).
- *Streptococcus pyogenes*
  - The cause of strep throat, rheumatic fever/heart disease, Scarlet fever, and more.
- Group B streptococcus (*streptococcus agalactiae*)
  - Colonizes vagina and is the most common cause of neonatal sepsis. Every pregnant woman should be screened for Group B strep.
- *Streptococcus pneumoniae*
  - Most common cause of bacterial pneumonia, meningitis, otitis media (children), and sinusitis. There are two vaccines for it (PCV13 and PPSV23), which are highly tested.
- All 4 clostridia (especially *C. difficile*)
  - *Clostridioides difficile* (*C. diff.* or *C. difficile*) is the most common cause of hospital-acquired diarrhea. It occurs when antibiotics kill off your good gut bacteria. The diarrhea is known to be super smelly (think: *C difficile* causes diarrhea whose smell is **difficult** to deal with).
- *Mycobacterium tuberculosis* (causes tuberculosis)
- *Mycobacterium avium*
  - A very important organism in AIDS patients (causes pneumonia and requires prophylaxis against when CD4+ count <50).
- *Pseudomonas aeruginosa*
  - Like S. *aureus*, can do a *ton* of different things.
- *Escherichia coli*
  - Found in feces and is a major cause of diarrhea. A commonly tested concept is that the *EHEC* subtype is found in undercooked hamburgers and can cause bloody diarrhea and hemolytic-uremic syndrome.
- *Borrelia burgdorferi* (Lyme disease)
  - If you see a bullseye rash, the answer is Lyme disease.
- *Treponema pallidum* (syphilis)
  - Know the 3 stages of syphilis, and that primary syphilis causes a *painless* genital lesion (chancre) with *painless* lymphadenopathy. Think: syphilis is painless.

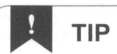

! TIP

Syphilis stages

1. Primary
Chancre (painless ulcer)

2. Secondary
Rash, condyloma lata (warty genital lesions)

3. Tertiary
Gumma (rubbery, granulomatous mass), neurosyphilis (tabes dorsalis, dementia), aortitis

- *Chlamydia trachomatis and Neisseria gonorrhoeae* (STDs)
- *Helicobacter pylori*
  - o Causes peptic ulcer disease (*'pylori'* is in reference to the pyloric sphincter of the stomach).

Viruses

- Herpes simplex virus 1 and 2
  - o Classically causes *vesicular* lesions.
- Varicella-Zoster virus
  - o Causes chicken pox and shingles.
- Hepatitis B and C
  - o Hepatitis can lead to cirrhosis and hepatocellular carcinoma. Especially understand Hepatitis B serologic markers (HBsAg, anti-HBs, etc.) and when each of these will be positive (see this chapter's *Tips and Key Concepts*).
- HIV
  - o Know *EVERYTHING* about HIV! *SUPER* high-yield.
  - o Especially know the main AIDS-defining illnesses/infections. There are many, but by far the most important and commonly tested are:
    - *Pneumocystis jirovecii* → **pneumo**nia
    - Cryptococcus neoformans → meningitis
    - Cryptosporidium → diarrhea
    - *Candida albicans* → esophagitis (**white** in color)
    - HHV-8 → Kaposi sarcoma
    - CMV → retinitis/colitis/esophagitis (think: cyto**mega**lovirus hits when your CD4+ count is **mega low** [<50])
    - Mycobacterium avium → Non-specific systemic symptoms
    - Toxoplasma gondii → brain abscesses

! TIP

The two 'crypto-' infections - Cryptococcus and Cryptosporidium - are in **alphabetical order**, in that Cryptococcus infects the head (higher) and Cryptosporidium infects the intestines (lower).

- Measles (rubeola) virus
  - o Especially know that measles causes Koplik spots (small, bluish-white spots in buccal mucosa).
- Influenza virus
  - o Especially understand the principles of antigenic drift and shift.
- Human papillomavirus (HPV)
  - o Responsible for most cases of cervical cancer (particularly subtypes HPV16 and HPV18). Also causes warts (HPV6 and HPV11).

Fungi

- *Candida albicans*
  - o Named *'albicans'* because it causes *white* lesions (e.g., yeast infection, oral thrush)
- *Pneumocystis jirovecii*

- o Is the first manifestation of AIDS in ~50% of cases. If you see pneumonia in an AIDS patient, assume it's *Pneumocystis jirovecii* unless given more information.
- The 4 systemic mycoses (for those in the US and/or those taking the USMLE) - namely, histoplasmosis, blastomycosis, coccidioidomycosis, and paracoccidioidomycosis.

Parasites

- *Plasmodium* (malaria)
  - o Pay particular attention to the pattern of fevers and to *Plasmodium falciparum's* complications (cerebral malaria, pulmonary edema, renal failure), as it's the deadliest species.
- *Toxoplasma gondii*
  - o Causes brain abscesses in AIDS patients (multiple ring-enhancing lesions).
- *Trichomonas vaginalis*
  - o Very commonly tested concept: know how to differentiate the 3 main vaginal infections – *Trichomonas vaginalis*, *Gardnerella vaginalis*, and *Candida albicans*. Simplified:
    - *Gardnerella*: just smells
    - *Candida*: just itches
    - *Trichomonas:* smells + itches

➤ Top resources

As discussed above, your top resources for microbiology are: **Sketchy Micro**, **First Aid**, and **YouTube**. While many students consider *Sketchy* far superior, an alternative resource is a book called ***Clinical Microbiology Made Ridiculously Simple***.

Clinical Microbiology Made Ridiculously Simple

A strong point of this book is that it's a far more casual read than most textbooks, which can take significant stress off learning this daunting subject. It also has lots of silly cartoons and illustrations that can help you understand and remember the information. Amazon has a *Look Inside* feature for the book's most recent edition, so take a peek inside to see for yourself if you'd like it.

➤ Useful YouTube videos & series

Series: USMLE Step 1 Drill Session [THE USMLE GUYS]

If you ever wanted a resource to review microbiology *passively* (e.g., when you're commuting or you just don't have the energy/motivation to actively study), the following are 3 videos that go through many microbiology questions and answers (no explanations – just questions and answers, one after the other).

➢ https://www.youtube.com/playlist?list=PLtVla_HPRH_uzF0DhhIlBKsEsFk-smzp8

Parasites: Protozoa (classification, structure, life cycle) [ATP]

Even if you're using Sketchy, this video provides a great overview of protozoa. While Sketchy does a great job of helping you remember the details of parasites, this video is superior in illustrating the "big picture". The same channel has 3 videos on helminths that can also be helpful, however this protozoa video is slightly higher in quality.

➢ https://www.youtube.com/watch?v=V4iSB0_7opM

Transformation, transduction, and conjugation (Horizontal Gene Transfer in Bacteria) [Henrik's Lab]

Really clear 5-minute video summing up bacterial gene transfer.

➢ https://www.youtube.com/watch?v=7tLV20dk-FM

DNA and RNA Viruses Mnemonic for USMLE Step 1 [Matt Skovgard]

If you're using Sketchy, this video is probably not necessary. However, if you're not, this mnemonic will be very helpful for remembering the categorization of viruses.

➢ https://www.youtube.com/watch?v=Df_qAFF58Ec&list=PLB1WoAapnStysgkmUMdQZ7A KHT-UdKybp

Taxonomy of Bacteria: Identification and Classification [Professor Dave Explains]

A good introduction and overview of the general principles around bacteria, including naming, staining, shapes, agars, and important characteristics.

➢ https://www.youtube.com/watch?v=8IJRzcPC9wg

Understanding Hepatitis B Serology Results [Zero To Finals]

A pleasant 10-minute explanation of the meanings of Hepatitis B surface, core, and envelope antigens and antibodies. Be sure to also see *Viruses* in this chapter's *Tips and Key Concepts* (page 133) to see useful mnemonics for these markers.

➢ https://www.youtube.com/watch?v=h_9EBVPADNE&ab_channel=ZeroToFinals

➢ Tips & key concepts

General

Classic WBC elevations:

- **Bacteria**: neutrophils
- **Viruses**: lymphocytes

- **Fungi**: lymphocytes
- **Parasites**: eosinophils

Bacteria

Bacterial genetics

1. **Conjugation**: two bacteria mating (*"conjugating"*) through a sex pilus; transfers a plasmid.

   o <u>Think</u>: *conjugal* partner (an unmarried couple).

2. **Transduction**: DNA transfer through a virus

   o <u>Think</u> of a *"transducer"*, which is any device that converts one form of energy into a readable signal. This should remind you that the signal (DNA) changes forms (from bacteria to virus to bacteria).

3. **Transformation**: bacterium picks up free-floating DNA and *transforms* itself with it.

Staphylococci and streptococci

Staphylococci **A** grow in clusters; streptococci **B** grow in chains.

- **Staphylococci → staff** meeting
- **Streptococci → "strip**tococci" (i.e., a long and narrow strip)

Syphilis blood tests

Examiners love to test on the diagnostic tests for syphilis. To make it very simple, there are 2 types of tests: **treponemal tests** (which, as the name implies, detect the actual *Treponema* bacteria) and **non-treponemal tests** (detect *antibodies* against *Treponema* rather than the actual bacteria).

- **Non-treponemal tests:** Since these detect antibodies, it takes around 3 weeks after infection for these tests to be able to detect syphilis (i.e., the time it takes to make enough antibodies). In other words, for the first 3 weeks after syphilis infection, the patient will test NEGATIVE using non-treponemal tests. Titers also will normally decline over time, and often become undetectable with successful treatment (= a negative test after treatment).
- **Treponemal tests:** Since these detect the actual bacteria, they can detect very early syphilis infection (<3 weeks). Treponemal tests remain positive for life.

The main tests you need to know are:

- Non-treponemal tests
    - o RPR (rapid plasma reagin)
    - o VDLR (Venereal Disease Research Laboratory)
- Treponemal tests

o   FTA-ABS (fluorescent **treponemal** antibody absorption test)

Dark-field microscopy is *not* used clinically.

Viruses

Positive vs. negative sense RNA viruses

What the heck does "positive-sense" and "negative-sense" even mean?! Well, it's actually a fairly simple concept: think of "sense" as whether the genetic information makes "sense" to the host or not. **Positive-sense RNA** is very similar to mRNA and can be immediately translated by the host cell, while **negative-sense RNA** is *complementary* to mRNA and thus must be converted to positive-sense RNA by an RNA polymerase before it's translated.

So, think of *positive-sense* RNA as RNA that *makes sense* to the host's ribosomes, and *negative-sense* RNA as RNA that *does not make sense* and must be converted into something that makes sense first.

Hepatitis B serologic markers

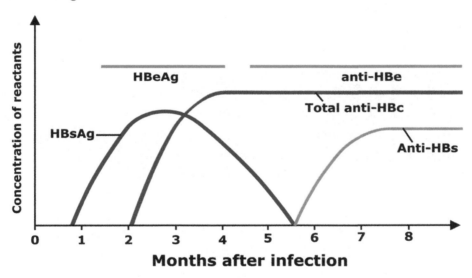

- The **SURFACE antigen** (HBsAg) and **antibody** (anti-HBs) are the most important markers and represent opposite ends of a spectrum. Presence of the surface antigen indicates **active infection** (= very bad); presence of the surface antibody hence represents immunity (= very good).
- Considering that **anti-HBs** is what gives immunity, it makes sense that hepatitis B immunization will give a person elevated anti-HBs and NOTHING ELSE! If the other antibodies don't confer immunity, why include it in the vaccine? On the other hand, if a person has recovered from a past infection, you'll see elevated anti-HBe and anti-HBc as well.
- **Envelope antigen** (HBeAg) indicates high transmissibility, and similarly, the antibody to it (anti-HBe) indicates low transmissibility. Just think about paper envelopes and mail –

whenever you want to transmit your mail, you need an envelope. No envelop means no transmitting your mail (i.e., hep B).

- Remember that **anti-HBc** may be the sole elevated marker of infection during the window period.

Parasites

Parasite classification

Parasites are divided into two main categories:

    A. **Protozoa**: single-celled
         o <u>Think</u>: **proto**type [i.e., it's a very basic type of parasite].
    B. **Helminths**: multicellular, worm-like parasites
         o <u>Think</u>: the more **hell**ish-looking parasites.

There are three types of helminths: cestodes **A**, nematodes **B**, and trematodes **C**. As they progress in alphabetical order, they become more and more round-looking and stubbier:

1. **Cestodes**: tapeworms.
2. **Nematodes**: roundworms.
3. **Trematodes**: flukes (leaf-shaped parasites).

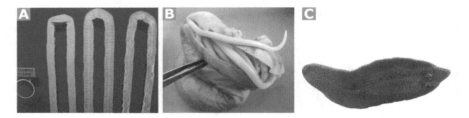

Ascariasis

Simply look at images of a**scari**asis and you'll forever think "a-**scary**-asis". *Ascaris lumbricoides* is the largest intestinal roundworm affecting humans, and it can grow so large that it causes intestinal obstruction **A**. It actually looks like a bowl of pasta **B**.

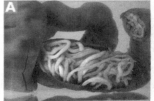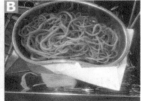

10. Immunology

Like biochemistry, much of the really fine details of immunology tend not to be particularly important for clinical practice in most specialties. Understanding general principles, however, like autoimmunity, vaccines, and immunoglobulin titers and isotype switching will benefit you wherever you go. As with biochemistry, immunology plays a more prominent role in certain types of lab-based medical research.

<u>Intensity</u>: medium-high

<u>Memorization</u>: 3/5

Some topics are very understanding-heavy (e.g., the various processes like inflammation, etc.), while some are very memorization-heavy (e.g., memorizing the different cytokines).

<u>Content emphasis on board exams</u>: low

➤ Approach & guidelines

Immunology is a subject in which you may encounter an extraordinary amount of detail, not all of which is essential or worthwhile for you to learn. For this reason, it's important to follow along with your *First Aid* book in order recognize what the *most important* concepts and facts are.

First Aid's immunology section is quite short and probably won't be sufficient for your immunology course, but it will serve you very well for the majority of your immunology content on board exams. Immunology is classically a lower-yield subject with a low reward:effort ratio. Therefore, it usually isn't necessary to look too deep into supplementary resources or textbooks.

There can also be great variance in terms of what your course actually tests you on. For this reason, your course lectures should play a more central role in guiding your studies. Try to find out from upper semester students what details your professor(s) like to test and what areas to pay more attention to. Typically, focusing on the highlighted/bolded information on your lecture slides rather than all the tiny details will be the most efficient use of your time (if your professor was kind enough to bold/highlight things…) Lastly, consider simply asking your professor what the most important information is for you to know from that topic – they'll very often direct you to the things they like to test without outright saying "this will be a question".

TIP

Rather than ask your professor, "What should we know from this?", ask "What's **most important** for us to know from this?" The former will likely get you an annoyingly unhelpful answer like, "Well, you should know everything…"(!)

A reasonable strategy for immunology may look something like this:

1. **Attend lectures**

    If your professor is good at teaching:

    - Learn the material from the lectures and follow along with your *First Aid* book.
    - At home, review your notes and lecture slides, and consider supplementing with an additional resource like YouTube videos or Google as needed.

    If your professor is NOT so good at teaching:

    - While in class, learn the same topic that's being taught via a commercial video series, YouTube videos, googling it, or using some other superior source
      - Preferably, study while sitting in the back of the class with headphones in. This way, you can keep an eye on what content your professor is emphasizing or spending a lot of time on. Alternatively, you can study elsewhere and find out from a classmate what was emphasized.
    - At home, review the lecture slides, and learn any details you didn't get to during class.
2. [OPTIONAL] Use **Sketchy Path** for immunodeficiency disorders.
3. **Do practice questions** (e.g., BRS, Kaplan) if you have any spare time remaining.

Immune processes

Immune processes like the inflammation and complement pathways, hypersensitivities, and T- and B-cell activation can be *very* confusing because of the sheer number of facts and the large amount of gibberish. *DO NOT* feel bad if it takes you a long time to understand them – this is normal.

What can help clarify these processes is to see them from different angles, i.e., watching different videos, reading different explanations, seeing different images, etc. to put all of the pieces together into a useful framework. The following processes are relatively high-yield, so try to learn them well:

1. Local inflammatory response
2. Arachidonic acid pathway
3. Hypersensitivities

Immunodeficiency disorders

Immunodeficiency disorders are one of the higher-yield topics within immunology. One good option for memorizing them is to use **Sketchy Path**. *Sketchy* works well for these disorders because they require a fair amount of brute memorization. Sketchy Path has four sketches for immunodeficiencies, which cover almost all of the important syndromes. Overall, these are useful and worth watching if you already have a Sketchy Path subscription, or plan to get one for pathology anyways. It is likely not worth buying a whole subscription just to watch them.

Other options are to learn the immunodeficiencies through commercial video series, YouTube videos, or even your lectures. Remember: follow along in and annotate your First Aid, as it contains an excellent chart in the *Immunology* chapter with almost all the major immunodeficiencies. In all honesty, you don't really need to know much more than what's in this table for board exams. It's just a matter of understanding this information so that you can remember it more easily.

Question banks

Given that immunology is a low-yield subject, whether or not you choose to run through practice questions should depend on how pressed you are for time.

Pressed for time

If you're concurrently studying a higher-yield subject like microbiology, pharmacology, pathology, etc. and you're concerned about your preparation for those, it's reasonable to forego completing immunology practice questions at this point (so long as you're adequately prepared to pass your school course). When you're reviewing all subjects at the end of your basic sciences (e.g., USMLE Step 1 prep time), completing the UWorld question bank will be more than adequate for immunology practice.

Not pressed for time

If you're not too pressed for time, consider completing the end-of-chapter quizzes in the **BRS Microbiology and Immunology** textbook. These not only do a good job of highlighting the highest-yield facts and concepts, but they're short questions, which means you can run through them fast (useful when first learning the subject). A USMLE question bank (e.g., Kaplan, Board Vitals) is another good option, but keep in mind their questions are longer so you may need more time to complete them.

➤ Top resources

As mentioned before, you don't really need to look deep into supplemental resources for immunology, aside from your usual First Aid, YouTube, and Google. If you already have a subscription to **Sketchy Path**, consider using it for the immunodeficiency disorders, as they can be very burdensome to remember. If you're not pressed for time, try to complete either **BRS Microbiology and Immunology's** end-of-chapter quizzes for immunology or some USMLE question bank immunology questions.

> ➤ **Useful YouTube videos & series**

Series: Inflammation [Armando Hasudungan]

Two thorough videos explaining the concept of inflammation.

➤ https://www.youtube.com/playlist?list=PLtVla_HPRH_vKNgQnCBd5LvTErQsXdX1m

Series: Hypersensitivity [Osmosis]

Excellent explanations of each type of hypersensitivity reaction.

➤ https://www.youtube.com/playlist?list=PLtVla_HPRH_sJ3IBguo06dez5jXT2_1NE

Chediak-Higashi vs. Chronic Granulomatous vs. Leukocyte Adhesion vs. Wiskott-Aldrich [Dirty Medicine]

An overview of 4 immunodeficiency disorders, discussing only the essential information, as well as some useful mnemonics. Check out the comment section, as people seem to be chipping in their own mnemonics.

➤ https://www.youtube.com/watch?v=MaOwZnSpkB4

Hypersensitivity | USMLE [Dirty Medicine]

A great overview of the 4 hypersensitivity types. Use this in conjunction with the Osmosis Hypersensitivity series mentioned above, which provides more in-depth explanations.

➤ https://www.youtube.com/watch?v=IpHaGrYNTag

Inflammatory Mediators [Dr. John Campbell]

Michael Caine-sounding professor discusses the prostaglandin/arachidonic acid pathway, as well as the inflammatory effects of prostaglandins, histamine, and cytokines. It's a bit long (22 minutes) and maybe not *as* essential as some of these other videos, but he's quite a good teacher and he can really help sharpen your understanding. Consider watching at x1.5 speed.

➤ https://www.youtube.com/watch?v=PE_D3Os7oWY

Inflammation – causes, symptoms, diagnosis, treatment, pathology [Osmosis]

Amazing overview of the inflammation process.

➤ https://www.youtube.com/watch?v=LaG3nKGotZs

USMLE STEP 1: Blood Transfusion Reaction w/ Questions [Randy Neil, MD]

AMAZING explanation of the types of blood transfusion reactions in under 5 minutes, followed by 7 minutes of working through questions.

➤ https://www.youtube.com/watch?v=7fbmgYg_EDU

Understanding the Cells of the Immune System [Zero To Finals]

A great video by Zero To Finals outlining the different types of immune cells.

➤ https://www.youtube.com/watch?v=9r0xzlpNjTw

Understanding the Immune System in One Video [Zero To Finals]

Brilliant overview of the immune system in 15 minutes. It obviously doesn't cover every detail, but it can help you develop a good mental framework of the immune system, which is really important given how confusing it can be.

➤ https://www.youtube.com/watch?v=_jBpv9fYSU4

➤ **Tips & key concepts**

MHC 1 vs. MHC 2

To remember that MHC 1 binds CD8+ cells and MHC 2 binds CD4+ cells, just remember that the lowest number is paired with the highest number (1 goes with 8).

Immunoglobulin isotypes

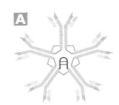

1. **IgM vs. IgG:** produced in response to infection
   o **IgM:** produced immediately ("**M**-ediately"); forms a pentamer 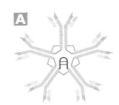, making it very large (looks kind of like a bunch of M's arranged in a circle; alternatively, think "**M** for **M**assive").
   o **IgG:** delayed production; small.

   This difference in size and production time between IgM and IgG is very important because it's the basis behind the pathology of **Rh alloimmunization**:

   ▪ In the first pregnancy, an Rh- mother produces IgM against her Rh+ fetus, but **IgM cannot cross the placenta** because of its size (= first pregnancy unharmed). In subsequent pregnancies, the mother will have IgG, which DOES cross the placenta and can attack and kill an Rh+ baby.

   You can also use IgM and IgG to tell whether an infection is **acute** or **chronic** (e.g., Hepatitis B titres).

2. **IgE:** activates **E**osinophils and mediates **E**nflammation in type 1 hypersensitivity.
3. **IgA:** **A**long mucous membranes (in secretions like tears, saliva, and mucus, and in GI tract).
4. **IgD:** **D**on't care (unclear function; forget about IgD).

Type 4 hypersensitivity

For whatever reason, the examples of type 4 hypersensitivity are quite commonly tested, so remember that **contact dermatitis** (including poison ivy and nickel allergies [e.g., jewelry or belt buckles]), **graft-versus-host disease**, and **PPD tests** all are type 4 hypersensitivies.

Blood transfusion reactions:

There are three main types of blood transfusion reactions (from fastest to slowest):

1. Anaphylactic
2. Acute hemolytic
3. Febrile nonhemolytic

The faster the reaction type, the worse the symptoms can be and the more potentially fatal it is.

Reaction	Timing	Symptoms	Memory Tip
Anaphylactic	Within minutes	Wheezing, hypotension/ shock, respiratory arrest	The timing makes sense: if you or anyone you know is allergic to something (e.g., cats, dust), how fast do they start sneezing when exposed to the allergen? Almost immediately!
Acute hemolytic (ABO mismatch)	Within 1 hour	Fever, hypotension, flank pain, tachycardia, hemoglobinuria, jaundice	The symptoms make sense when you simply think about hemolysis - the hallmark of this reaction. Hemolysis causes jaundice from release of bilirubin from RBCs. Flank pain and hemoglobinuria occur because the products of ruptured RBCs are toxic to the kidneys. Tachycardia and tachypnea occur because this is an antibody-mediated reaction, and the antibodies promote inflammatory cytokine release.
Febrile nonhemolytic	1-6 hours	Fever, headache	This reaction is mild because as its name implies, it's not even hemolytic! It's simply a bit of fever that comes on gradually. You don't even really have to do anything about it – it self-resolves in 15-30 minutes.

Transplant rejection

- **Remembering pathogenesis:** the key to remembering the pathogenesis for hyperacute, acute, and chronic transplant rejections is to focus on the **timeline**, which happens to be implied in their names. Graft-versus-host disease (technically not a type of transplant rejection) has variable timing, but the name itself literally tells you the pathogenesis (graft T cells in the transplanted bone marrow or stem cells attack the host's organs).

- **Remembering features:** All three transplant rejection types (hyperacute, acute, and chronic) involve blood vessels. The key to differentiating them is again to focus on the **timeline**. The faster the reaction is, the faster the blood vessels get occluded/damaged.

Transplant rejection types

Type	Timing	Pathogenesis	Features
Hyperacute	Within minutes	Pre-existing recipient antibodies attack donor antigen (type 2 hypersensitivity) • Makes sense: the only possible way you can get a reaction within *minutes* is if the antibodies are already formed.	Widespread thrombosis • Makes sense: immediate closing off of vessels causes immediate (hyperacute) rejection.
Acute	Weeks to months	T cells react directly to the donor organ (e.g., forming new antibodies) • Makes sense: it takes weeks to form new antibodies from scratch.	Vasculitis • Acute inflammation of vessels (vasculitis) takes longer than thrombosis but not as long as fibrosis and smooth muscle proliferation (chronic rejection).
Chronic	Months to years	T cells respond to the host's own APCs that are presenting donor peptides • Chronic rejection is like acute rejection except it involves an extra step (the APCs have to process and display the antigen) – hence it makes sense that it's the slowest.	Vascular smooth muscle proliferation and fibrosis • Proliferation and fibrosis are very slow processes!

Serum sickness vs. Arthus reaction

Both serum sickness and the Arthus reaction are type 3 hypersensitivity reactions that occur after being given a drug or vaccine. Differentiating the two is as simple as asking "is the reaction local or systemic?"

- Local → Arthus reaction
- Systemic → **Serum** sickness (the name literally tells you the reaction is disseminated all throughout the **serum**)

NOTES

11. Psychiatry

In addition to being a basic science subject, psychiatry is one of the core rotations of your clinical years. Most of the psychiatry you learn during your basic sciences will directly benefit you in the psychiatry core. Furthermore, even if you're not a psychiatrist or a family doctor, a basic level of psychiatric knowledge is relevant to most specialties in order to rule out psychiatric causes for a patient's symptoms. You may commonly also need to manage patients with comorbid psychiatric illness.

Intensity: medium

Memorization: 3/5

Grasping the different disorders and knowing how to differentiate between them is understanding-heavy. Diagnostic criteria, minimum durations for diagnosis, and treatments must simply be memorized.

Content emphasis on board exams: high

➤ Approach & guidelines

Psychiatry is a relatively straightforward subject in that there aren't many tiny, hidden details that you have to worry about. No chromosomes, biochemical pathways, histological findings, etc. Simply knowing the disorder's symptoms/findings, duration, treatment, and any major associations mentioned in First Aid will suffice to score you most points in board exams. In fact, it's fairly safe to say that if you know and truly understand the material in First Aid's psychiatry chapter (which is quite short) and annotate a few missing details and disorders, you should be on track to do very well. Most of these missing details may come from a major question bank (e.g., UWorld, Kaplan).

Therefore, don't spend much time reading big textbooks on psychiatry. With that said, differentiating between disorders and remembering timelines and associations can sometimes be tricky, so practice questions are very beneficial for reinforcing your memory and understanding.

The recommended approach to learning psychiatry is:

1. Learn the subject through **class lectures** OR a **video lecture series** while following along in and annotating your *First Aid*.
2. Complete a major **question bank**'s psychiatry questions.

It generally really is that simple. Don't overcomplicate it!

> Top resources

As mentioned, all you really need is your *First Aid* book and a USMLE question bank. If your class lectures are not great, you can use a video lecture series. If you don't have one, you can use a psychiatry course on YouTube created by MadMedicine! – Education (listed in *Useful YouTube channels*), which should be *more than* sufficient.

> Useful YouTube channels

MadMedicine! – Education

MadMedicine! – Education has an excellent psychiatry course that is on YouTube in full. This course can serve as a free alternative to a commercial video series.

> https://www.youtube.com/playlist?list=PL2-kln7xNP6s5M29jXRkBWJPRyIOuxvvt

> Useful YouTube videos & series

Series: USMLE STEP 1: BEHAVIORAL SCIENCE [*Randy Neil, MD*]

This is a series of 4 videos in which Dr. Neil walks you through answering high-yield psychiatry questions. Consider this if you need extra help with the following 4 topics: childhood psychiatric disorders, defense mechanisms, personality disorders, and psychotic vs. mood disorders.

> https://www.youtube.com/playlist?list=PLtVla_HPRH_sGEHgc6QD7j1uP_n1_mIEj

> Tips & key concepts

Childhood disorders

- The CLASSIC sign of Shaken Baby Syndrome is retinal hemorrhages (extremely important - you MUST know this!)
- Rett syndrome → regression. Also, picture a young girl named Rett sending you a text message saying "XD" (the squinting-eyes laughter emoji) to remember Rett syndrome is X-linked dominant, and that the syndrome occurs almost exclusively in females.
- Tourette syndrome: symptoms > 1 year
  - Mnemonic: you have to wait so long to diagnose it because you want to see if the child is just messing with you and trying to get away with swearing (note: this is probably not the real reason!).

Adult disorders

Schizo- timeline

Just remember two numbers – **1 month** and **6 months**.

- **Brief** psychotic disorder: < 1 month
    - The name literally tells you it's the **briefest** one.
- Schizophren**iform** disorder: 1-6 months
    - *"Schizophreniform"* means it's **"like schizophrenia"**, but it's not quite schizophrenia. The schizophrenia is still **form**ing.
- Schizophrenia: **> 6 months**
    - Pronounce it "**SIX**-ophrenia".

Schizotypal personality disorder

- Think: "**atypical**" (dresses weirdly, eccentric/magical thinking)

Manic vs. hypomanic episode

To help remember the 4 major differences between the two, just think: manic is worse and more serious in every way.

1. Manic episode lasts ≥ 1 week (vs. ≥ 4 days for hypomanic episode)
2. Manic causes impairment (vs. no marked impairment in hypomanic)
3. Manic may cause hospitalization (vs. hypomanic, which will NEVER)
4. Manic may have psychotic features (vs. hypomanic, which will NEVER)

Borderline personality disorder

Splitting is a major defense mechanism.

- Think: *splitting* something into two sides is literally what an actual *border line* does. Therefore, the disorder is characterized by a person standing on a borderline (metaphorically), in that it's very easy for them to flip-flop between two clearly separate sides.

Malingering vs. factitious disorder

Malingering is faking illness for external gain (e.g., compensation), while factitious disorders are for internal gain (e.g., sympathy).

- Think: Malingering does not have the word *"disorder"* in it. This is because it's not a disorder – it's just lying to obtain something of value. Factitious *disorder* is a disorder, meaning they get some sort of psychological comfort from the attention.

Anorexia nervosa vs. bulimia nervosa

The main difference between anorexia nervosa and bulimia nervosa is that anorexia has low body mass, whereas body mass is normal in bulimia.

- o <u>Think</u> of the word "**an**orexia" – the *"an-"* means *absent* or *without* (i.e., body mass).

Agoraphobia

Agoraphobia is a fear of places perceived as difficult to escape from (e.g., <u>public spaces</u>, crowds, closed spaces, public transportation).

- o <u>Think</u>: in **ago**raphobia, patients don't want to *ago* anywhere.

Phencyclidine intoxication

Phencyclidine intoxication (PCP, a.k.a. Angel Dust) classically presents with **violence**. If you see a question on a drug intoxication causing a patient to be violent, the answer is most likely PCP.

- o <u>Think</u>: it should really be called "*Devil* Dust"
- o <u>Think</u>: *Angel* Dust causes nystagmus, so picture the patient looking around at hallucinatory *angels*.

12. Physiology

Physiology is one of the "Big 3" subjects, along with pathology and pharmacology. These subjects form the core of your basic sciences and comprise most board exam questions. They're also highly important to your practice as a physician. Physiology, in particular, significantly deepens your understanding in medicine, and will prove highly useful in ways that you will likely grow to appreciate.

Intensity: high

Memorization: 1.5/5

Content emphasis on board exams: high

> **Approach & guidelines**

Find good explanations

The *BRS Physiology* textbook (along with its end-of-chapter quizzes), *First Aid*, and your school's lecture slides together can serve as an effective roadmap and checklist to ensure you're covering the most important concepts in physiology. However, as you might have guessed, physiology is extremely understanding-oriented. In practice, this means initially getting thorough explanations of concepts through your lectures, a commercial video series, YouTube videos and Google. Not only will they help you understand the logic behind the concept, but they will also tend to highlight the key take-away points (as not all information is equally important!)

You can either quickly skim through your review resources (BRS and *First Aid*) first and then proceed to your explanatory sources, or vice-versa. The order is a matter of personal preference.

Draw or write out pathways

Whenever you're learning a pathway (e.g., a hormone production pathway), practice writing it out in very simple terms several times. After a few times (with spaced repetition), it *will* stick. For example:

Renin-angiotensin-aldosterone system

Angiotensinogen ——→ Angiotensin 1 ——→ Angiotensin 2 ——→ Aldosterone and ADH
       [Renin]   [ACE]

Give special attention to enzymes that are acted on by drugs (e.g., in the renin pathway, ACE is inhibited by ACE inhibitors). You can note this with color coding or by adding a comment.

Visualization

Use vivid imagery to work out and understand principles wherever possible. It's an invaluable technique that will not only help the concept stick with you in the long term, but will also deepen your understanding of physiology and medicine altogether. This is particularly important in cardiovascular and respiratory physiology, as they involve macroscopic processes that are more easily visualized.

Explain things out loud

Explaining physiological concepts and processes to yourself or someone else does three very beneficial things: it helps you understand the concept better by forcing you to present it in simple, logical terms; it identifies your areas of confusion or misunderstanding; and, it strengthens your memory of the concept. If you don't want to literally explain it out loud, it is still effective to explain it in your head.

Equations

Respiratory, renal, and cardiovascular physiology, in particular, have multiple equations to learn. **The more complex the equation is, the less likely it is that you will be asked to actually plug in values and calculate something with it.**

For example, you should expect to see a question that gives you stroke volume (SV) and heart rate (HR) and asks you to calculate cardiac output ($CO = SV \times HR$), or that gives you minute ventilation (V_E) and physiologic dead space (V_D) and asks you to calculate alveolar ventilation ($V_A = V_E - V_D$). On the other hand, while such equations are in your *First Aid*, it is highly unlikely that you'll be asked to actually calculate something like a gas' diffusion rate using Fick's law ($V_{gas} = A \times D_k \times ([P_1 - P_2]/ T)$), or pH using the Henderson-Hasselbalch equation ($pH = 6.1 + \log([HCO_3^-]/0.03PCO_2)$) on standardized exams. Therefore, don't waste time practicing these calculations.

In any case, the most important part of any equation in physiology – simple or complex – is **understanding the general principle behind it**. In other words, know what happens to one particular variable if another variable increases or decreases, and by what factor. For example, if tidal volume increases, what happens to physiologic dead space (as seen in the equation $V_D = V_T \times [PaCO_2 - P_ECO_2 / PaCO_2]$)? If a blood vessel's radius doubles, what happens to the flow rate through it (as seen in the equation $Flow = \pi P r^4/8nl$)? Understanding these relationships are your priority.

Question banks

As one of the "Big 3" subjects, and due to the large amount of information (of differing importance) – it's really important to complete a physiology question bank.

Your top two choices are **BRS Physiology** (end-of-chapter quizzes) and a USMLE question bank (e.g., Kaplan, UWorld). For first-time learners, *BRS Physiology* questions are highly recommended, given their short, rapid-fire nature. Ideally, you should aim to complete the *BRS* questions and then do as many USMLE question bank questions as you can with the remaining time you have. For those returning to physiology for dedicated review, **UWorld** is the gold standard.

> **Top resources**

Books

BRS Physiology

As discussed previously, a great physiology review book many students like to use is **BRS Physiology**. It is quite concise (around 300 pages) and does a pretty good job of leaving out unnecessary details. The end-of-chapter quizzes are especially useful. If you're not a fan of this book, at least do the quizzes. They're particularly good for when you're first learning the subject because they're short questions that test the most important concepts in physiology and leave out unnecessary details, such as the patient's age, past medical history, etc. Those long vignettes you see in UWorld or Kaplan question banks are great practice for board exams like the USMLE and MCCQE, but the shorter BRS questions help you learn the bread-and-butter of the subject faster, and hence may be better earlier on.

Commercial video series

Any of the big 4 courses (Kaplan, Boards and Beyond, DIT, Lecturio) will work fine, however **Boards and Beyond** and **Kaplan** might be your best choice. Both series have been highly praised by students, and Kaplan's Dr. Conrad Fischer is quite lively and animated, which has made his lectures quite popular amongst students. It is also worth considering another excellent and highly-praised course:

Physeo

Physeo has a style similar to Pathoma – the narrator presents and explains simple slides and uses drawings or images to visually demonstrate the concept. Their website has some sample videos to check out (www.physeo.com/physiology/), as does their YouTube channel (see *Useful YouTube channels*).

Websites

TeachMePhysiology (www.teachmephysiology.com)

One particularly useful website to use as a supplementary resource for certain topics is www.TeachMePhysiology.com. Just like TeachMeAnatomy, it covers most high-yield topics in a clean format, with great explanations and emphasis on high-yield information and clinical correlates.

> ## Useful YouTube channels

Armando Hasudungan

Armando Hasudungan is very effective in explaining physiology. What's nice about his explanations is that they tend to be quite thorough and touch on important details other channels might skip over - all while still being easy to follow and not overly long.

> ➢ https://www.youtube.com/user/armandohasudungan

Dr. John Campbell

Dr. John Campbell has a ton of videos on physiology concepts (see his playlists for the one on physiology, which currently has 24 videos). He's a good teacher and these may be useful as a reference for some topics you need extra help with. Sometimes his pace can feel a little bit slow, in which case consider playing them at x1.5 speed. Regardless, his videos are still way shorter than Dr. Najeeb's.

> ➢ https://www.youtube.com/c/Campbellteaching

Physeo – USMLE Step 1 Prep

As mentioned in *Top Resources*, Physeo has an excellent video series for physiology, and a few of these videos are on their YouTube channel (see link).

> ➢ https://www.youtube.com/playlist?list=PLfJxXWqsLMw95dogaWkYhb6LHAKNtiSrl

> ## Useful YouTube videos & series

Cardiovascular

Cardiac Conduction System and Understanding ECG, Animation [Alila Medical Media]

Nice explanation of the cardiac conduction system, the basic EKG waveform, and the relationship between the two.

> ➢ https://www.youtube.com/watch?v=RYZ4daFwMa8

Electrocardiography (ECG/EKG) – basics [Osmosis]

A clear and easy-to-follow explanation of how an EKG works and what the different "leads" are.

> ➢ https://www.youtube.com/watch?v=xIZQRjkwV9Q

Heart Murmurs and Heart Sounds: Visual Explanation for Students [Zero To Finals]

Explains the reasoning behind why the various murmurs sound the way they do.

> https://www.youtube.com/watch?v=wYZbMoWjLEg

Endocrine

Hypothalamic Pituitary Thyroid Axis (regulation, TRH, TSH, thyroid hormones T3 and T4 [Armando Hasudungan]

A review of the production and feedback cycles of TRH, TSH, and T3/T4 in <5 minutes.

> https://www.youtube.com/watch?v=KzM8BiSnKQM

Review of Thyroid Physiology – Endocrinology | Lecturio [Lecturio]

A pleasant little review of thyroid function tests (TSH, T3, and T4) and their interpretations in under 3 minutes.

> https://www.youtube.com/watch?v=8MRddajuMcg

Physiology of Insulin and Glucagon [Strong Medicine]

Explanation of the synthesis and effects of insulin and glucagon, as well as the effects of GLP-1, GIP, amylin, cortisol, growth hormone, and epinephrine on blood glucose.

> https://www.youtube.com/watch?v=-3J6QRMerQE

Gastrointestinal

Physiology Basics: The Digestive System, Animation [Alila Medical Media]

A nice 4-minute overview of GI physiology for when you're first starting out.

> https://www.youtube.com/watch?v=zSXgoYdHotw

USMLE Step 1 Intro to Hormones [Physeo – USMLE Step 1 Prep]

Explanation of the functions of CCK and secretin, including a few questions. Unfortunately, the other hormones are only available on their website via subscription.

> https://www.youtube.com/watch?v=rmvrFPTkjSY

Musculoskeletal

Neuromuscular Junction, Animation [Alila Medical Media]

A nice animation and explanation of the neuromuscular junction (<5 minutes) if you needed a refresher.

> https://www.youtube.com/watch?v=zbo0i1r1pXA

Muscles, Part 1 - Muscle Cells: Crash Course A&P #21 [CrashCourse]

An engaging refresher on muscle physiology (actin-myosin coupling, etc.) in 10 minutes by CrashCourse, if you needed it. Most of this will be repetition, so consider playing at x1.5 speed or skipping parts. Skip the first minute and 10 seconds (not much info).

➤ https://www.youtube.com/watch?v=Ktv-CaOt6UQ

Neurology

Blood Brain Barrier, Animation [Alila Medical Media]

A pleasant 4.5-minute animation of the blood brain barrier.

➤ https://www.youtube.com/watch?v=noWwbvmdhL0

2-Minute Neuroscience: Blood-Brain Barrier [Neuroscientifically Challenged]

Another pleasant 2-minute overview of the blood-brain barrier (may be helpful in reinforcing a better mental image of it).

➤ https://www.youtube.com/watch?v=e9sN9gOEdG4

Renal

Nephrology – Physiology Reabsorption and Secretion [Armando Hasudungan]

A thorough, yet concise (13 minutes) video on where different ions, urea, water, etc. are secreted or reabsorbed in the nephron, and what transporters they use.

➤ https://www.youtube.com/watch?v=ko_XD4jPEo8

Acid/Base || USMLE [Dirty Medicine]

Helps you determine whether a set of lab values shows acidosis or alkalosis, and whether it's respiratory or metabolic.

➤ https://www.youtube.com/watch?v=J9jisOXB_Oo

Anion Gap EXPLAINED [HippocraTV]

An invaluable video that clarifies a really confusing and high-yield concept – high anion vs. normal anion gap acidosis – in under 7 minutes.

➤ https://www.youtube.com/watch?v=sQnEFVNrY74

Renin-Angiotensin-Aldosterone System [susannaheinze]

A really good, visually appealing explanation of the renin-angiotensin-aldosterone system. It even covers the drugs that inhibit each step.

➤ https://www.youtube.com/watch?v=qTPqjDD0vhY

Reproductive

Understanding the Menstrual Cycle [Zero To Finals]

An amazing video explaining the menstrual cycle in under 10 minutes.

➤ https://www.youtube.com/watch?v=3Lt9I5LrWZw

Respiratory

Respiratory Gas Exchange [Armando Hasudungan]

Armando explaining the transport of oxygen and CO_2 in the blood.

➤ https://www.youtube.com/watch?v=qDrV33rZlyA

Respiratory System Physiology – Ventilation and Perfusion (V:Q Ratio) Physiology [Armando Hasudungan]

A beautiful explanation of V:Q ratios. Highly recommended.

➤ https://www.youtube.com/watch?v=-mL_NQ3pKnA

Understanding Spirometry – Normal, Obstructive vs Restrictive [Armando Hasudungan]

Another great video by Armando on spirometry and FEV_1/FVC ratios in obstructive and restrictive lung diseases.

➤ https://www.youtube.com/watch?v=YwcNbVnHNAo

➤ **Tips & key concepts**

Cardiovascular

Radius of a blood vessel (Poisseuille's equation)

Board exams LOVE to test the relationship between the radius of a blood vessel and the blood flow through it – namely, that **flow is proportional to radius to the power of 4 (r^4)**. This means that doubling the radius of a vessel increases flow by 16 times.

This is so commonly tested because it relates to IV lines, organ perfusion, and other critical topics. You almost certainly will be tested on the relationships between the variables in this equation (*especially* radius). The two most common questions are:

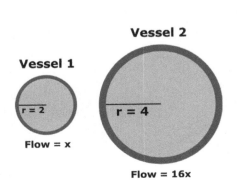

Vessel 2

Vessel 1

r = 2

r = 4

Flow = x

Flow = 16x

- *"Which of the following variables will have the greatest impact on flow rate?"*
  - Answer: radius

- *"The radius of the blood vessel (or IV catheter) is doubled (or halved) – how will the flow rate change?"*
  - Answer: multiple/divide by 16.

Murmurs

- Heart murmurs **radiate toward where the blood is flowing**. The two classic radiations that you must know are:
  - **Aortic stenosis**: radiates to the carotids.
    - Makes sense, since the carotids branch off the aorta.
  - **Mitral regurgitation**: radiates to the axilla.
    - The mitral valve is tilted anteroposteriorly, so blood flow in mitral regurgitation is aimed up and posteriorly.

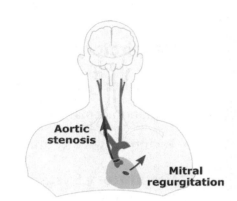

- Additional tips:
  - The **smaller the hole, the *louder* the murmur**. This means that more severe ASDs and VSDs are actually *quieter*. Picture a garden hose: the smaller you make the diameter (by squeezing it), the more explosively the water comes out.
  - Regurgitation murmurs sound "**blowing**" in quality.
  - The one murmur that originates entirely *outside of the heart* (**patent ductus arteriosus**) is also the one murmur that is *continuous* (i.e., throughout systole and diastole).
    - This is because there's always some blood moving through arteries, so there's always a pressure gradient from the aorta to the pulmonary artery.
  - Tricuspid regurgitation: <u>think</u> "they've probably **tri**-ed **drugs**" (tricuspid regurgitation is associated with infective endocarditis from **IV drug use**).
  - Mitral murmurs: think "**rheu-mitral**" (**mitral** valve damage has an extremely important association with **rheumatic** fever).
    - Note: mitral valve damage caused by rheumatic heart disease starts as mitral *regurgitation* and later progresses to mitral *stenosis*.

- S3 vs. S4 heart sounds:
  - **S3**: sounds like "**Tri**cycle" (S1 ["tri-"], then a gap, then S2 and S3 ["-cycle"] close together).
    - Bonus: picture a very chubby kid on the tricycle to remember S3 represents ventricular overfilling (e.g., heart failure).
  - **S4**: sounds like "Foramen" ("**Four**amen") (S4 and S1 ["fora-"] close together, then a gap, then S2 ["-men"]).

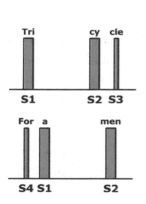

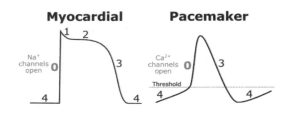

Myocardial vs. pacemaker action potential upstrokes

- **Myocardial:** Na^+ channels (think: *myo* → *so*[dium])
- **Pacemaker:** Ca^{2+} channels (just think 'the other one')

Endocrine

C-peptide is a part of proinsulin (insulin precursor) and will always be produced with endogenous insulin production. *Exogenous* insulin lacks C-peptide.

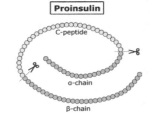

o This is really important because it can tell you if a person has intentionally induced hypoglycemia (i.e., factitious disorder).

Gastrointestinal

GI hormones

When learning the functions of GI hormones, remember to **think about the name** of the hormone to remember at least one of their functions, and **think about protagonistic actions** to make sense of any other functions.

For example, secretin helps with the digestion of food once it reaches the duodenum – hence all of its functions should relate to food digestion in the duodenum (e.g., secretion of bicarbonate, decreasing gastric acid secretion, and increasing bile secretion).

- **Gastrin:** stimulates **gastric** acid secretion, increases **gastric** motility, stimulates growth of **gastric** mucosa.
    - o Gastrin is all about when food is in the **stomach** (*"gastric" = stomach*). **Gastric acid secretion** happens when food is in the stomach obviously. It therefore makes sense that gastrin also **increases gastric motility**. Since it stimulates the parietal cells of gastric mucosa to secrete acid, it makes sense that gastrin also causes **growth of gastric mucosa**.
- **Somatostatin:** *decreases* gastric acid/pepsinogen, pancreatic secretion, gallbladder contraction, and insulin/glucagon release.
    - o Somato**statin** causes **stasis** of the GI system (i.e., it inhibits anything to do with food digestion).
- **Cholecystokinin (CCK): gallbladder contraction**, sphincter of Oddi relaxation, increases pancreatic secretions.
    - o *Cholecysto* = gallbladder; *kinin* = movement → tells you it causes **gallbladder contraction**. It thus makes sense that CCK also stimulates **sphincter of Oddi relaxation** (the sphincter through which bile comes out into the duodenum). Since the gallbladder secretes bile into the duodenum to help digest food, this tells you CCK's work revolves around food being in the duodenum. Hence it also functions to **increase pancreatic secretions** (which get secreted through the very

same sphincter!)
- **Secretin:** stimulates **secretion** of bicarbonate and bile, decreases gastric acid secretion.
  - o Just like CCK, secretin is all about helping digest food once it's in the duodenum. The duodenum is not the stomach – you need to tone down the acidity. Hence secretin increases pH by **stimulating secretion of bicarbonate** and **decreasing gastric acid secretion**. Again, since secretin deals with digesting food when it's in the duodenum, it also **increases bile secretion**.
- **Ghrelin:** increases appetite.
  - o <u>Think</u>: **Ghrelin** causes stomach **ghrumbling** (alternative: "*Ghrrrr...hungry*" [like when you become "hangry"]).
- **Motilin:** stimulates gastric and small intestine **motility** (produces migrating motor complexes).
- **Vasoactive intestinal polypeptide (VIP):** relaxes smooth muscles both in blood vessels (= **vasodilator** → hence increases intestinal water and electrolyte secretion) and in the intestinal wall/sphincters.
- **Glucose-dependent insulinotropic peptide (GIP):** stimulates **insulin** release.
- **Pepsin:** **pep**tide (protein) digestion.
- **Intrinsic factor:** vitamin B12-binding protein (brings vitamin B12 **into** the body).

Hemotology

Coagulation cascade

- PTT has more letters in it, so it corresponds to the pathway with more numbers (intrinsic pathway). PT has fewer letters, so it corresponds to the pathway with fewer numbers (extrinsic pathway).
- Mnemonic to match PT/PTT to the words 'intrinsic'/'extrinsic':
  - o **PT - Play Tennis** (you play tennis outside = extrinsic)
  - o **PTT - Play Table Tennis** (you play table tennis inside = intrinsic)
- Warfarin vs. heparin:
  - o **Warfarin:** primarily affects extrinsic pathway.
    - ▪ <u>Think</u>: **war** is extrinsic (you don't go to war intrinsically...)
  - o **Heparin:** primarily affects intrinsic pathway.
    - ▪ <u>Think</u>: the other one

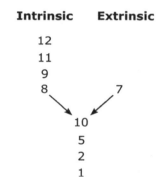

Renal

Glucose is osmotically active

It's really important to know that **glucose is osmotically active**. This means that if you have glucosuria, you will lose water with it because water will follow the glucose across the glomerular epithelium into the nephron, and you'll pee it out. This is why major hyperglycemia can cause severe dehydration (seen in hyperosmolar hyperglycemic state and diabetic ketoacidosis).

Most diuretics cause hypokalemia

All diuretics, aside from "potassium-sparing diuretics", can cause hypokalemia. This is because they all work by increasing sodium excretion. When the sodium reaches the collecting duct, some of it gets exchanged for potassium via the **Na+/K+ pump**.

> o This is important for both exams and real life because hypokalemia and hyperkalemia can cause serious arrhythmias.

Acid-base physiology

Acid-base physiology is one of, if not, the most important concept in renal physiology.

Ensure you know how to determine whether an acid/base derangement is respiratory/metabolic acidosis or alkalosis, and whether it is compensated or not. You WILL get plenty of questions on this, and you WILL see this in real life. Follow these two steps to determine what kind of disturbance it is *quickly*:

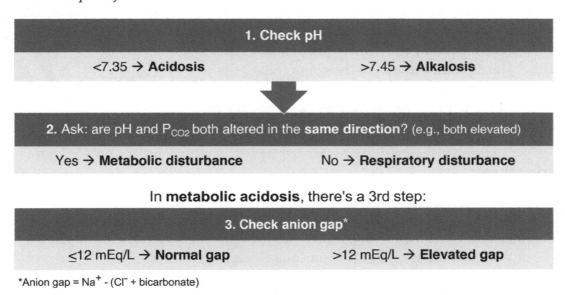

Renal clearance

To remember the equation for renal clearance ($C_x = U_x V/P_x$), think *"UV over P"*, and picture someone peeing (P) under the sunlight (UV).

Filtration/clearance patterns of substances

Make sure you know the filtration and clearance patterns of **creatinine, inulin, glucose,** and **para-aminohippuric acid (PAH)**:

1. **PAH: PAH**sses right through your kidneys (100% excretion of all PAH that enters kidneys). Hence, PAH clearance provides an estimate of effective renal plasma flow (eRPF).

2. **Inulin**: is **indolent** – it's freely filtered but is neither reabsorbed nor secreted. Hence, its clearance is used to calculate glomerular *filtration* rate (GFR).

3. **Creatinine**: *almost* the same as inulin, hence its clearance can give an approximation of GFR. However, it slightly overestimates GFR because creatinine is **secreted** a little by the renal tubules. Think: creatinine is a waste product so obviously you'd like to secrete it rather than reabsorb it.

4. **Glucose**: should normally not be in the urine at all, as it is completely reabsorbed in the proximal convoluted tubule (PCT). When plasma glucose becomes >200 mg/dL (i.e., diabetes), the Na^+/glucose cotransporters that reabsorb it become saturated and can't reabsorb any more – hence you get glucosuria.

Juxtaglomerular apparatus

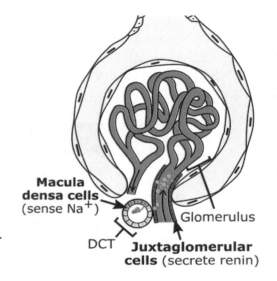

- Macula **densa**: salt **sensa**
  - ○ Macula densa cells are **NaCl sensors** in the wall of the distal tubule. When they sense low NaCl, they signal to the juxtaglomerular cells to increase renin secretion.
- **Juxtaglomerular** cells: **juxtaposed** to the **glomerulus**
  - ○ As implied by the name, these cells are juxtaposed (beside) to the glomerulus (specifically, they are smooth muscle of the afferent arteriole). It thus makes sense that they function to **secrete renin** directly into the blood.

Reproductive

Estrogen synthesis

- Cholesterol is converted to **androgens** via desmolase in **theca cells**; stimulated by LH
  - ○ Think: "**Theca** cells make your muscles **theca** (thicker)".
- Androgens are converted to **estrogen** via **aromatase** in granulosa cells; stimulated by FSH
  - ○ Think: "**Arom**atase creates the **aroma** of a woman (estrogen)".
  - ○ Think: FSH: "**F**emale **s**timulating **h**ormone" (and just remember LH as being the opposite, i.e., stimulates androgens).

Menopause marker

The most specific lab marker of menopause is **FSH**. This makes sense because the problem in menopause is a decline in the number of *follicles* – hence the body secretes a ton of *follicle*-stimulating hormone to try to stimulate the follicles.

Corpus luteum

- **Lutein**izing hormone (LH) surge leads to corpus **luteum** creation (i.e., ovulation).

- Think of the **corpus** luteum as the **corpse** of the follicle. Once the egg gets released from the follicle, you're just left with a corpse. This corpse still tries to help out its old friend, the egg, by secreting progesterone and estrogen so that the egg may be able to implant and grow in the uterus (were it to get fertilized).

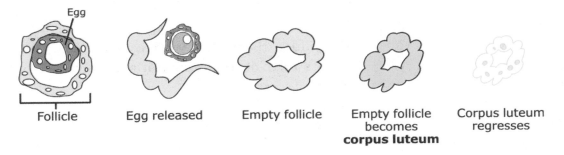

Menses

Menses is caused by a fall in progesterone.

- ○ Think: **Progesterone** is **pro-gestation** – in other words, it maintains the endometrium to support implantation. Hence it makes sense that when progesterone decreases sharply, the endometrium dies off (= menses).

Fertilization

Most common site of fertilization: **ampulla** of the fallopian tube.

- ○ Think: pregnancy gets **amped** up in the **ampulla.**

Human placental lactogen

Human placental lactogen (unsurprisingly, produced by the placenta) stimulates insulin production and increases insulin resistance.

- ○ Think: The word **lacto**gen should remind you of **lactose** – a sugar – which tells you it deals with insulin.

Testosterone

- Dihydrotestosterone (DHT): Think of DHT as the hormone in males that does **amazing things early on** and **terrible things later**.
  - ○ Early: differentiation of penis, scrotum, and prostate
  - ○ Late: prostatomegaly, balding
- Remember that **5α-reductase** is the enzyme that converts testosterone to dihydrotestoserone because the name "**dihydro**testosterone" literally tells you it's testosterone that has been **reduced** by receiving **two hydrogen ions**. This is an important enzyme, as you can inhibit it with finasteride to treat benign prostatic hyperplasia.

Respiratory

O_2 vs. CO_2 diffusion

An extraordinarily important concept is the idea that **CO_2 diffuses across the alveolar wall much more easily (x20) than oxygen**. This means that even if you have lung scarring (e.g., COPD), you can still regulate your $PaCO_2$ just fine so long as your respiratory effort and circulation are intact. The CO_2 can still diffuse. Therefore, if you see an increasing $PaCO_2$ in a COPD patient, this is a very big deal as it's a sign of **respiratory fatigue**. Your PaO_2 on the other hand may be *expected* to decrease with lung scarring.

O_2 vs. CO_2 balance

Remember that oxygenation is NOT your only concern – you also need to closely regulate CO_2. The effects of both high and low CO_2 are serious (high → acidosis; low → alkalosis). This means that in conditions that cause persistently low blood oxygen (COPD, high altitude, and pulmonary embolism), you're at risk for respiratory alkalosis via hyperventilation. Your body is conflicted – it needs more oxygen, but by hyperventilating, it makes your blood CO_2 lower and lower.

13. Pharmacology

Pharmacology is one of the "Big 3" subjects (the others being physiology and pathology). These are the core of your basic sciences, and they comprise most board exam questions. They're also highly important to your practice as a physician. Even if particular drugs are not commonly prescribed in the specialty you're hoping to practice in, their side effects and interactions could be relevant.

Also, as a doctor, people outside of work may often ask you about their medications, so you should have at least a basic understanding of them!

Intensity: high

Memorization: 5/5

Content emphasis on board exams: high

➤ Approach & guidelines

Pharmacology is in many ways similar to microbiology. It contains general principles that you must learn, followed by a big list of items (in this case, drugs) with non-intuitive names that you have to memorize. Therefore, similar strategies can be used.

As with microbiology, supplementary resources are critical. Unless your professor is an excellent teacher and your lecture slides are great, consider starting off by learning the subject through supplementary resources, and return to your slides in order to review for your school exams.

The subject can be divided into two parts: **learning general principles** and **memorizing drugs**. Start off with learning general principles *first*.

1. Learning general principles

Overall approach

First Aid's Pharmacology chapter covers most of the important topics in general principles that are tested on by the USMLE step 1. If you're ever pressed for time, just make sure you know the content in First Aid thoroughly and you should be prepared for roughly 75-80% of Step 1 questions on pharmacology general principles.

In addition to *First Aid*, you have three main options to round out your knowledge and get more detailed explanations: (1) class lectures, (2) a review book, or (3) a commercial video series. If you're pressed for time and your class lectures are decent, just stick with your lectures alone – you'll have to study them anyways for your school exams.

If you have time or your lectures are poor, you can add a commercial video series or a review book (*Lippincott: Pharmacology* or *BRS Pharmacology*). See *Top resources* on page 164 for a review of these.

Additional strategies

Autonomic receptors and their effects are very high-yield. Take the time to learn them well the first time around – not only are they heavily tested on, but they will come up again and again throughout your basic sciences. Sketchy does an excellent job teaching autonomic receptors, especially with their sympathetic sketch. These sketches are fairly dense and they'll take some time to go through, but it'll be a wise investment for your future.

Remember to **think about the meanings of the words** when learning new pharmacologic terms, as they're usually very descriptive. For example, bioavailability is the fraction of administered drug that actually ends up being available to your body (i.e., that reaches systemic circulation unchanged).

2. Memorizing drugs

Overall approach

The following combination should leave you more than well-prepared for learning drugs:

First Aid   +   Sketchy Pharmacology   +   1 supplement

Choices for supplements include:

- Your class lectures (your top choice if they're good quality)
- A good Anki deck
- A traditional flashcard deck (Lange Pharmacology Flashcards or Pharm Phlash!)
- A USMLE question bank (e.g., UWorld, Kaplan).

Note: If your class lectures are effective, just stick with them as your supplement! This will save you time, since you will have to study them to prepare for your school exams anyways.

See '*Top resources*' (page 164) for a breakdown of some of these resources. See '*How to use Sketchy*' in the Microbiology chapter (page 126) – Sketchy Pharm is used exactly the same way.

Sketchy alternative

Sketchy Pharm, like Sketchy Micro, is an exceptional resource, and it is highly recommended that you use it to memorize your drugs. However, if you're simply not a fan and want an alternative, consider either a textbook (**Lippincott: Pharmacology** or **BRS Pharmacology**), a video review course (Kaplan specifically has received praise from students, but any of the 4 main courses will do), or increasing your reliance on Anki/flashcards and supplementing them with YouTube videos.

Drug suffixes

Most of the time, agents within the same drug class have a common suffix. For example, ACE inhibitors end in '-*pril*' (e.g., lisinopril, captopril), and local anesthetics end in '-*caine*' (e.g., lidocaine, benzocaine). Make it a priority to learn these suffixes. It will allow you to recognize drugs within that class without necessarily having to memorize each individual agent.

To memorize suffixes:

1. Use Sketchy Pharmacology
   o Sketchy usually incorporates the suffix into their sketch.

   OR

2. Create your own mnemonics
   o Think of a word that sounds like the suffix, and then relate that to the drug's function or action. For example, picture your tongue going **numb** after licking a candy **cane** to remember that **local anesthetics** end in '-**caine**'.
   o *First Aid* has a page that contains all major drug suffixes and their classes in their pharmacology chapter. Use this page to assist you as you progress through the subject.

Additional strategies

Think of any new drug you're learning in terms of three things:

1. **Mechanism of action**
2. **Clinical use**
3. **Side effects**

The connection between the mechanism of action and the clinical use is often obvious or better explained (e.g., a vasodilator that's used to treat hypertension). Many side effects, on the other hand, might seem a little more random. As much as possible, try to **find a connection between the mechanism of action and the side effects** to help make them more intuitive instead of just memorizing a list of random side effects. For example, it makes sense that cholestyramine – a bile acid sequestrant – can cause fat-soluble vitamin deficiencies, as less bile means less absorption of fat. Sometimes there won't be any obvious connection, but when there is, it'll be beneficial to your memory to think about them.

For some drugs, you'll come across a side effect that is very unique and that few or no other drugs have. Pay especially close attention to these, as they're not only exam favorites, but they also sometimes make the question a dead giveaway. For example, if a question mentions *"orange sweat"* or *"orange tears"*, you can immediately be nearly certain the question is talking about *rifampin* – the classic medication associated with orange body fluids.

> **Top resources**

Sketchy Pharmacology

Sketchy Pharm, like Sketchy Micro, is excellent. Their sketches cover most of the information you need to memorize for medications, including mechanism of action, clinical uses, and side effects. They make the information both easy to remember and enjoyable to learn. One weakness of this visual approach is that sometimes the mechanism of action is better understood and remembered through simple writing rather than symbols. Some sketches are also a bit too crowded. However, despite these weaknesses, Sketchy Pharm is still highly recommended. It doesn't have to be all or nothing – use Sketchy for whatever drugs you find useful and skip whatever you dislike and supplement it with another resource or form of learning.

You can consider Picmonic (a similar sketch-based learning website) as an alternative, but in all honesty the quality of Sketchy is far superior.

Anki (flashcard app)

Since Anki allows you to do rapid-fire repetition of information, it can be very useful for pharmacology, which is a very memorization-heavy subject. You can either make your own decks or download a pre-made one off of Reddit. To find pre-made decks, a simple Google search will do the trick.

Traditional flashcards

If you're considering buying a flashcard deck, you have two top choices:

Lange Pharmacology Flashcards

This is generally going to be your top choice, as it is specifically geared towards medical school (in particular, the USMLE Step 1). It has 260+ flashcards.

Pharm Phlash!

Although this is a popular flashcard deck, it is geared towards nursing students. Most of the information is still the same, but it also contains clinical practice advice that you do not need to know as a basic science medical student.

Use Amazon's *Look Inside* feature to see which of these two decks you can envision yourself using for many hours.

Books

As discussed previously, a textbook is generally not necessary. However, if you'd like to use one, your top two choices are:

Lippincott Illustrated Reviews: Pharmacology

This book has been widely praised and recommended. It is easy to read, has a pleasant layout, and contains lots of images and graphs. It is a bit lengthy at ~580 pages though.

BRS Pharmacology

An advantage of BRS over Lippincott is that it is shorter, at ~380 pages. The information is in bullet points, so some might prefer the paragraph-style writing of Lippincott.

Both books contain a *Look Inside* feature on Amazon.

Websites

Pharmacology2000 (www.pharmacology2000.com)

Pharmacology2000 is a website that contains a *ton* of free medical pharmacology questions. Some questions are beyond the scope of the basic sciences (e.g., routes of administration, complex drug interactions), but many are still useful. Overall, this website can be a useful supplement, and you should consider at least checking it out.

➤ Useful YouTube channels

Dirty Medicine

As with other subjects, Dirty Medicine does a good job of not only explaining concepts, but also highlighting the highest yield information for board exams. He also presents a lot of helpful mnemonics. If you're using Sketchy to learn drugs, this channel is not necessary, but it can help if you need clarification. He currently has 18 pharmacology videos – see the following playlist:

➤ https://www.youtube.com/playlist?list=PL5rTEahBdxV6kvrOR0aL9Su4V40OJs8LH

Speed Pharmacology

Speed Pharmacology is a wonderful channel that has excellent, visually appealing videos that outline the mechanisms of drugs, though they don't cover clinical uses or side effects. If you're not using Sketchy, you should definitely watch some of these. However, even if you are using Sketchy, these can be great adjuncts because they provide clear breakdowns of the mechanisms of action in ways Sketchy cannot.

➤ https://www.youtube.com/channel/UC-i2EBYXH6-GAglvuDIaufQ

➤ Useful YouTube videos & series

Series: Pharmacokinetics [Handwritten Tutorials]

A wonderful series of five videos (5-7 minutes each) explaining pharmacokinetics (absorption, distribution, metabolism, and excretion) and relevant terms and formulae you must know, like clearance, volume of distribution, etc.

➤ https://www.youtube.com/playlist?list=PLzl4lgX_3RvdGiqSs3hmmUdWEAqL3dEY7

Antibiotic Classes in 7 minutes!! [Dr Matt & Dr Mike]

A well-organized 7.5-minute overview of all the main antibiotic classes and their mechanisms of action, as well as whether they target gram positive or negative bacteria. This video has a high benefit:time ratio.

➤ https://www.youtube.com/watch?v=gqoqexfqoBM&t=77s

Enzyme Kinetics with Michaelis–Menten Curve | V, [s], Vmax, and Km Relationships [PremedHQ Science Academy]

A nice 10-minute video fir those needing some clarification on Michaelis-Menten curves and concepts like Km and Vmax. It does not discuss Lineweaver-Burk plots though.

➤ https://www.youtube.com/watch?v=kmyR1cYxRL4

Pharmacology – ADRENERGIC RECEPTORS & AGONISTS (MADE EASY) [Speed Pharmacology]

As discussed earlier, it's really important for you to know the effects of the different adrenergic receptors very well. This is a great 18-minute explanation by Speed Pharmacology, and it includes the most important agonists.

➤ https://www.youtube.com/watch?v=KtmV-yMDYPI

Pharmacology – PHARMACODYNAMICS (MADE EASY) [Speed Pharmacology]

A 13-minute explanation of important pharmacodynamics concepts with nice visuals. It covers receptor types (ligand-gated ion channels, G protein-coupled receptors, enzyme-linked receptors, intracellular receptors), EC_{50} and EC_{max}, agonists/antagonists, and therapeutic index.

➤ https://www.youtube.com/watch?v=tobx537kFaI&t=9s

> **➤ Tips & key concepts**

General Principles

Pharmacokinetics vs. pharmacodynamics

Pharmacokinetics is what your body does to the drug (e.g., how it absorbs, distributes, metabolizes, and excretes it), while **pharmacodynamics** is what the drug does to your body (e.g., mechanism of action, effects on organs). To remember the former, think of *kinesiology* or *kinetic energy* to remember 'kinetic' means 'relating to motion'. To remember the latter, either simply think "the other one", or think of social *dynamics* to remind you that it deals with mechanisms and effects.

Michaelis-Menten vs. Lineweaver-Burk plots

Think of the curves in the letter 'm' to remember that michaelis-menten plots are curved (hyperbolic), while Lineweaver plots, as the name hints, are linear.

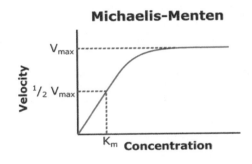 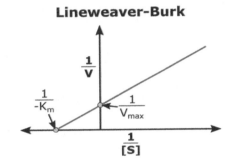

Efficacy vs. potency

Use these two words in a sentence to help you remember their meanings.

- **Efficacy:** for example, "I'm a more *effective* worker than him" implies you can have a *greater overall effect* at the task then this 'him' fellow. This should help you remember that efficacy is about the **maximal effect of the drug (V_{max})**.
- **Potency:** for example, "Careful! That spice is really *potent!*" implies you only need a *tiny amount* of spice to light your tongue up. This should help you remember that potency is about the **amount of drug needed** for a given effect.

Drug elimination (zero vs. first order)

- **Zero-order elimination** gives **zero** cares about the drug concentration (i.e., *constant rate of drug elimination* regardless of its concentration). This means if you take a large amount of these drugs (like in an overdose), it will take a long time to eliminate them (= bad!). Remember the 4 most important examples of zero-order drugs by thinking: 2 CNS drugs (phenytoin and ethanol) and 2 blood drugs (aspirin and warfarin).

 TIP

Technically, it's called "zero-order" because when you put any number to the **power of zero (x^0)**, the result is always the same: 1 (i.e. it's constant). Similarly, zero-order elimination is constant.

- **First-order elimination** is simply "the other one" (i.e., rate of elimination is *directly proportional to the drug concentration*). Most drugs have first-order elimination ("*1st* order = the #1 elimination method").

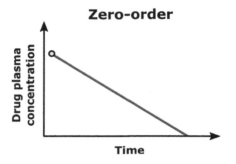

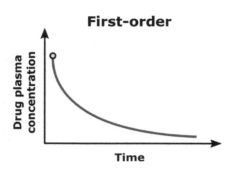

Ions

- Ions (charged particles) love water and hate lipid.
- This means they can't cross lipid barriers well, while neutral substances can. This helps you remember two important principles:
  1. **Charged particles tend to have a low volume of distribution (V$_d$).** In other words, an ionized drug stays mostly in the blood stream and doesn't diffuse much into your tissues.
  2. **Renal excretion of acidic or basic drugs speeds up by adding agents with the OPPOSITE pH** (i.e., ionizing the drug). This is key, for example, in treating an overdose.
- Ionizing the drug causes it to become trapped in the urine, unable to be reabsorbed by the kidney.
- Therefore, treat *weak acids* with **bicarbonate** to make the urine more *basic*, and treat *weak bases* with **ammonium** chloride to *acidify* the urine.

Key side effects

The following are the highest-yield side effects in pharmacology, which you MUST know (you *will* see questions on most, if not all, of these):

Antibiotics

- **Vanc**omycin: Red-Man syndrome (think: **VanGogh**-mycin, and picture Van Gogh painting a red man).
- Tetracyclines: teeth discoloration in children (think: after taking tet**racyclin**e, your teeth will need *recyclin'*), teratogen (sounds like *tetracycline*).
- **Clin**damycin: *Clostridium difficile* infection (or, think: **clin**damycin **cleans** out the good bacteria from your gut, allowing *C. difficile* overgrowth).
- Aminoglycosides: ototoxicity, acute tubular necrosis, neuromuscular blockade, teratogen.
- **Fluoro**quinolones: tendon/cartilage damage (think: **fluoro**quinolones make your tendons/cartilage delicate as a **flower**).

- Rifampin: orange body fluids (picture the rust on an old **rifle**).
- Ethambutol: red-green color blindness (think of it as etham**beautiful** to remember it makes you lose the ability to see the **beautiful** colours of red and green).

Antineoplastics

- Metho**trex**ate: mucositis, pulmonary fibrosis
  - <u>Think</u>: when you go on long **treks**, your lips get dry/cracked and you become out of breath.
- Bu**sulf**an: pulmonary fibrosis, hyperpigmentation
  - Remember hyperpigmentation by remembering that **sulf**ur is a *pigmented* substance (it's yellow).
- Cyclophosphamide: hemorrhagic cystitis
  - Picture a **cyclone** of blood in your bladder.
- Anthracyclines (Doxorubicin): dilated cardiomyopathy (which is prevented with Dexrazoxane).
  - Picture the heart as a giant **ruby** ("doxo**ruby**cin")
- Paclitaxel, Vincristine/Vinblastine: peripheral neuropathy
  - Picture **Pac**-Man (**pac**litaxel) eating your peripheral nerves
- Trastuzumab: cardiotoxicity
  - "It's hard to **trust** someone after they've **broken your heart**".

Autonomics

Anticholinergics: know the whole anticholinergic syndrome (decreased sweating/hyperthermia, blurry vision, dry mouth, delirium/confusion). *Especially* know that the risk of CNS effects (confusion, agitation, delirium) are much higher in the **elderly**, hence you must prescribe them with caution.

Blood & inflammation

- Heparin: Heparin-induced thrombocytopenia (causes thromboembolism – NOT bleeding!).
- Warfarin: hypercoagulability in the *early* period (hence requiring heparin "bridging").
- Statins: myopathy
  - <u>Think</u>: statins destroy your fat (i.e., cholesterol) but they can also destroy your muscle.
- Niacin: cutaneous flushing/warmth (antidote = NSAIDs)
  - <u>Think</u>: Niacin warm (i.e., *"nice and warm"*)
- NSAIDs: peptic ulcer disease, GI bleeding

Cardiovascular & renal

- ACE inhibitors: angioedema, cough (caused by bradykinin – avoid by using angiotensin-2 receptor blockers [ARBs] instead).
- Acetazolamide: proximal renal tubular acidosis

- o Think: **acid**azolamide
- Loop diuretics: ototoxicity (your ears are **loop**-shaped!).
- Spironolactone: antiandrogen effects (e.g., gynecomastia)
  - o Think about the "*-lactone*" part of spironolactone. It should remind you of *lactation* (i.e., antiandrogen effects).
- Calcium channel blockers: heart failure worsening
  - o Makes sense – calcium channels facilitate muscle contraction. Thus, blocking them in arterial smooth muscle is great (decreases blood pressure), but not so great in the heart if there's already some heart failure (weakens an already ineffective pump).
- Nitroprusside: cyanide toxicity
  - o Think: nitroprus**syanide**
- Beta **blocker**: impotence & heart block (it's not called a beta **blocker** for nothing).
- Nitrates: life-threatening hypotension if used with Viagra (sildenafil) (both are vasodilators).
- Digoxin (**digital**is): yellow vision
  - o Think: **digital** monitors sometimes have color display problems.
- Amiodarone: blue/gray skin
  - o **Amio-darone**: Picture your **Amigo** colouring his skin blue/gray because you **dared** him to.

Endocrine

- Corticosteroids: Cushing's syndrome (know all the symptoms – e.g., buffalo hump, moon facies, abdominal striae).
  - o Corticosteroid inhaler: oral thrush (prevent by rinsing after use).
- Senna: melanosis coli (harmless but commonly tested because it looks scary).
- Metformin: lactic acidosis
  - o "Met**formin** be *formin'* lactic acid"

Neurology & psychiatry

- Barbiturates: severe CNS depression, respiratory/cardiovascular depression (possibly fatal).
- Benzodiazepines: dependence
- Triptans: coronary vasospasms
  - o **Trip**tans make your coronary arteries start **trip**pin' out).
- Inhaled anesthetics: malignant hyperthermia (treated with dantrolene)
  - o Picture those fire breathers who put fuel in their mouths and breath out fire (except with inhaled anesthetic instead of fuel).
  - o **Dantrolene**: picture **Dan** *throwin'* water on a patient who's burning up.
- Opioids: respiratory depression (can be fatal) (antidote: naloxone).
  - o **Naloxone**: think "*no relaxing*" (i.e., wakes you up).
- SSRIs: sexual dysfunction, serotonin syndrome

- o <u>Think</u>: *Serotonin* gives a man **zero tone in** his private part…(technically, delayed orgasm is more common, but erectile dysfunction can happen too).
- Tricyclic antidepressants: <u>C</u>onvulsions, <u>C</u>oma, <u>C</u>ardiotoxicity (the "3 C's")
- MAO-inhibitors: hypertensive crisis with tyramine-containing foods (aged cheese, wine).
  - o Picture dictator **Mao** really disliking aged cheese and wine and getting agitated when he's served them.
- Lithium: Ebstein anomaly (congenital heart defect)
- Valproic acid: neural tube defects, pancreatitis
- Carbamazepine: diplopia, teratogen
  - o Diplopia: You know how cars can sometimes look like they have faces because of their headlights? Picture a **car's** (**car**bamazepine) headlights being *cross-eyed.*
  - o Teratogen: Getting hit by a **car** in pregnancy will obviously harm the baby.
- Phenytoin: diplopia, gingival hyperplasia (**funny**toin makes your gums look **funny**), teratogen, **mega**loblastic anemia (<u>think</u>: **mega funny**!)
- Typical antipsychotics: extrapyramidal symptoms (treated with benztropine), neuroleptic malignant syndrome (treated with dantrolene and bromocriptine)
  - o Just like with inhaled anesthetics, picture your **Bro** (**bro**mocriptine) and **Dan throwin'** (**dan**trolene) water on a patient who's burning up (that's a good *bro* right there).
- Clozapine: agranulocytosis
  - o Clozapine is a gold-standard treatment when other antipsychotics have been ineffective. But it's not used as 1st line treatment due to these serious side effects. Hence, <u>think</u>: there's a reason you keep **Cloz**apine in the **closet**.
  - o Additionally, <u>think</u>: **cloz**apine keeps your granulocytes in the **closet**.
- Risperidone: hyperprolactinemia
  - o <u>Think</u>: **risper**ries (raspberries) go well with **milk** (not really though, but just go with it).

NOTES

14. Pathology

Pathology is the highest-yield subject in your basic sciences. As a doctor, even if particular diseases are not directly under the umbrella of your specialty, their complications are often still relevant. You very well may also have to manage patients with comorbid diseases, and you should have a decent understanding of those diseases and how they affect the patient's overall management.

<u>Intensity</u>: high

<u>Memorization</u>: 2/5

<u>Content emphasis on board exams</u>: *very* high

> ➤ **Approach & guidelines**

Overall approach

In learning pathology, there are some things that you absolutely MUST do, some things that are highly recommended, and some things you can consider:

MUST-*do*

Pathoma (video lecture series)

Highly recommended

At least two of these three question banks:

- **Robbins questions** (*"Robbins and Cotran Review of Pathology"*)
- **WebPath questions** (FREE, really memorable, and has lots of pictures)
- **USMLE question bank** (e.g., *Kaplan, UWorld*).

These are recommendations for question banks to do *while first learning pathology*. Regardless of what you choose here, remember that every student should eventually complete the UWorld question bank before moving on from the basic sciences.

Consider

- **Rapid Review Pathology** (textbook) by *Edward Goljan*

   Often simply called "Goljan", this book has been widely praised for being a good review book. However, in all honesty, First Aid generally suffices as a review book for pathology, especially if you annotate it. Nonetheless, you can look into Goljan to see if it's something that would work well for you.

- **Robbins Pathology** (textbook)

  The Robbins textbook can be useful as a *reference* book for certain concepts that you need more clarification with. It's really only worth considering if your school/library already has it (i.e., it's not worth buying). It's far too long to just sit and read the whole thing (it's almost 1000 pages).

- **Sketchy Path**

  Sketchy Path should only be used for details that require pure memorization. Do NOT use it for the bulk of your pathology learning, as it's really important to actually understand pathology and not just memorize. With that said, Sketchy Path can be fairly helpful for memorizing disease facts like:

  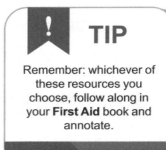

  ! TIP

  Remember: whichever of these resources you choose, follow along in your **First Aid** book and annotate.

  - o Inheritance patterns
  - o Chromosome numbers
  - o Autoantibodies in autoimmune diseases (e.g., anti-smooth muscle, etc.)
  - o Tumor markers (especially for leukemias and lymphomas)
  - o Other disease associations

See the *Top Resources* heading for a breakdown of each resource.

Study plan

Before starting pathology, read the *Tips and key concepts: Golden general principles* part of this chapter (page 178). This will give you a good foundation for pathology that you can apply to any organ system.

Subsequently, when studying each particular organ system, a solid approach is to:

1. Skim through that system's pathology section in *First Aid* to get a general idea of what you're going to learn.
2. Read the *Pathognomonic features* and *Specific tricks and mnemonics* for that system in the *Tips and Key Concepts* section of this chapter.
3. Go through the Pathoma lectures for that organ system, following along in and annotating your *First Aid*.
4. Go through your class' lecture slides/notes.
5. [*OPTIONAL*] Refer to the *Robbins* textbook if you need clarification, and to Sketchy Path if you need help remembering details that require pure memorization.
6. Complete *Robbins* and WebPath questions for the system; with whatever time you have leftover, do USMLE question bank questions (e.g., Kaplan, UWorld).

Note: It's also reasonable to do questions right after completing that system's Pathoma lectures rather than waiting until the end. See which works better for you.

Buzzwords

A huge mistake when studying pathology is to rely on memorizing 'buzzwords' without understanding what they mean. Buzzwords are catchy words or phrases that are supposed to describe a classic disease finding. While buzzwords might have scored you lots of exam points in the past, standardized exams have evolved significantly. Nowadays, it's more common for exams to describe the actual *meaning* of the word rather than to use the word itself.

For example, "*bamboo spine*" is a buzzword for the classic x-ray finding of widespread vertebral blunting and fusion in ankylosing spondylitis, such that the spine loses its curvature and looks really straight – like bamboo. On a standardized exam though, instead of saying "bamboo spine", they might say something like "diffuse ossification of the intervertebral discs and loss of curvature" and expect you to know they're talking about ankylosing spondylitis.

In fairness, this ends up being better for your learning, as it forces you to actually learn concepts rather than blindly memorizing words you don't understand.

Ultimately though, you should still definitely learn the buzzwords for two reasons:

1. They are excellent **memory cues** for the actual concept (they tend to be very visually descriptive) and for the disease as a whole (i.e., they may be pathognomonic), and
2. Your **school exams** might still use them.

The point is: also **know the concept behind the buzzword!**

Pathognomonic features

"*Pathognomonic*" means a sign or symptom that is **distinctively characteristic of a certain disease**, i.e., if a pathognomonic feature is seen, the disease is present. Pathognomonic features are extremely valuable because once you've learnt them, you immediately know what the diagnosis is any time you hear them. Therefore, any time you see a pathognomonic or highly unique feature of a disease, be sure to learn it very well, and take your sweet, delicate time if needed! See *Tips and key concepts: Pathognomonic features* (page 185) for a list of these features.

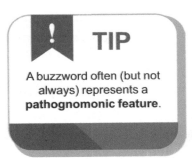

! TIP

A buzzword often (but not always) represents a **pathognomonic feature**.

> **Top resources**

Video courses

Pathoma

Pathoma is a video lecture series by Dr. Husain Sattar, who does a truly outstanding job in explaining pathology in a way that really makes sense. It's this element of "making sense" and genuinely understanding why things are the way they are that is so helpful in remembering pathology long-term. It also does an excellent job in highlighting general principles that recur all throughout pathology.

As mentioned previously, Pathoma is a *MUST* for pathology. Just buy it.

Pathoma has a corresponding book called Fundamentals of Pathology that is automatically included with the Pathoma subscription. It contains bullet points of the information in the lectures. Consider referring to it, but remember that by far the most important element of Pathoma is the lectures.

Books

Rapid Review Pathology (aka Goljan)

As mentioned previously, this book is an option for pathology review for those who prefer something more detailed than their First Aid book. It is quite lengthy, at around 860 pages. It's written in bullet-point form, which some might like or dislike.

Question banks

Robbins and Cotran Review of Pathology ("Robbins Questions")

Robbins questions have been widely praised as an excellent question bank for learning pathology. Most of its questions are not entirely standardized exam-style (e.g., USMLE, MCCQE) but rather shorter, more direct questions. This is especially advantageous for when you're first learning the subject, as it removes all the "fluff" and makes your learning more time-efficient. The fifth edition contains 2000 multiple choice questions along with explanations.

Tip: try to read (or at least skim through) the explanation for every question, even if you answered it correctly. You'll often still learn something new!

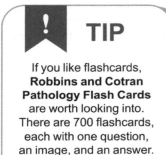

! TIP

If you like flashcards, **Robbins and Cotran Pathology Flash Cards** are worth looking into. There are 700 flashcards, each with one question, an image, and an answer.

WebPath (webpath.med.utah.edu/)

Their nearly three-decade old website might appear primitive, but *WebPath* is truly an *amazing* free learning resource for pathology. The site has two main features: a **teaching section** and a **question bank**.

The teaching section (*"General Pathology"* and *"Systemic Pathology"*) is excellent and quite unique in that their teaching revolves around images. Each topic (e.g., "thromboembolism"), has several images, and with each image there's a short explanation of the fact or principle being taught. This makes the learning very visual and quick, and you can run through them almost like flash cards.

The question bank (*"Examinations"*) contains a ton of questions neatly arranged by topic and organ system.

> ## Useful YouTube channels

Dirty Medicine

Dirty Medicine's pathology videos can be useful to check out if you'd like a nice one-video recap of all major diseases in a particular topic (e.g., lung tumors, nephritic/nephrotic syndromes, etc.), or you're looking for mnemonics. See the following playlist:

> https://www.youtube.com/playlist?list=PL5rTEahBdxV7HBl0eT7T7BgYNsilHZucL

Larry Mellick

Larry Mellick is perhaps the best channel on YouTube for showing real hospital cases. He does an outstanding job talking you through the disease and/or procedure as you watch the real thing. This can be super helpful in remembering a certain element of a disease that might otherwise not be sticking too well in your mind, as seeing a disease manifestation is usually more memorable than reading it.

> https://www.youtube.com/user/lmellick

MedCram – Medical Lectures Explained CLEARLY

MedCram gives lectures on a ton of different diseases through KhanAcademy-style presentations (i.e., drawing/writing on a black screen). It would probably be better to just stick with Pathoma, but this channel might be helpful for any topics not covered by Pathoma or that you simply need clarification with.

> https://www.youtube.com/channel/UCG-iSMVtWbbwDDXgXXypARQ

Osmosis

Osmosis can be a nice complement to your primary sources for any diseases you need more help understanding or that you'd like a more visual explanation of. Be aware that Osmosis sometimes goes into more detail than required for your basic sciences.

> https://www.youtube.com/channel/UCNI0qOojpkhsUtaQ4_2NUhQ

Paulthomasmd – Dr. Paul

Similar to Larry Mellick, Dr. Paul is a useful channel for seeing some real pediatric cases. He usually gives good explanations of the condition and its management as well.

> https://www.youtube.com/user/paulthomasmd

> ## Useful YouTube videos & series

There's an immense number of topics in pathology, and it's more feasible to simply refer to the aforementioned channels and search for what you need.

> ➤ **Tips & key concepts: Golden general principles**

The following are some of the highest-yield principles in pathology. These will keep recurring over and over all throughout your basic sciences and well beyond. It is recommended that you read ALL of these before you start learning pathology. Consider returning to them every now and then, as you'll see them in a new light as your knowledge progresses.

Cardiovascular

Blockage of an artery leads to ischemia. Blockage of a vein leads to edema.

- o   Remember: veins have fenestrations (tiny gaps in the walls), so when there's a pressure buildup, fluid seeps out into the surrounding tissues (= edema).

The "Big 4" cardiovascular risk factors

The "Big 4" things that damage the walls of arteries are:

1. Smoking
2. Hypertension
3. Diabetes
4. Hyperlipidemia

The right side of the heart is much more compressible than the left side.

This makes sense, as the left heart deals with much higher pressures and must pump harder, which make its walls thicker.

- o   This is important because when something compresses the heart (namely, pericardial effusion/tamponade and tension pneumothorax), the cause of cardiovascular collapse is **improper diastolic filling** rather than systolic dysfunction. This restricted filling manifests as dilated neck veins.

Decreased oxygen to any tissue leads to arterial vasodilation EXCEPT in the lung.

In any other tissue, vasodilation of arteries occurs more blood can get to the ischemic tissue. In the lung though, segments not getting much oxygen from ventilation have their arteries *vasoconstricted* because the job of the lung is to oxygenate blood. Why would you want to perfuse a segment of lung that's not going to be able to oxygenate your blood? Instead, the incoming blood diverts to regions receiving more oxygen.

Though this is advantageous for oxygenating your blood, the downside is that it can lead to **cor pulmonale** – right-sided heart failure from pulmonary hypertension.

Thromboembolism

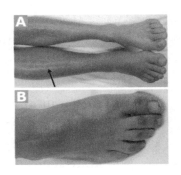

- **Venous** thromboemboli start as deep vein thromboses 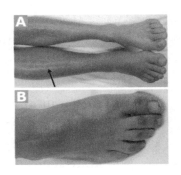 (DVTs), usually in the leg, and go to the lung (= pulmonary embolism).
- **Arterial** thromboemboli usually start in the heart (from some turbulent flow or stasis – usually atrial fibrillation, myocardial infarction, or a mechanical valve) and usually go to the brain (= stroke) or leg (= acute ischemia).

Infection & Inflammation

Chronic inflammation of a tissue can lead to neoplasm.

A tissue that's being chronically irritated needs to continuously proliferate to repair itself from the damage and keep remodeling to become more resilient. If this happens long enough, the cells can start to become more and more funky (*hyper*plasia/*meta*plasia → *dys*plasia → *neo*plasia).

Chronic inflammation of tissues generally causes deposition of fibrous tissue (fibrosis).

This happens because your body is trying to protect itself from a continuous irritant by repairing itself with a more sturdy material. The problem is, that irritant isn't going away, so the fibrosis keeps on building and building. Ultimately, if the irritant persists long enough, this fibrosis can lead to organ dysfunction.

Some prominent examples of this include:

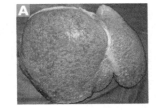

- Various autoimmune conditions and inhaled irritants (e.g., asbestos, coal dust) leading to lung fibrosis (interstitial lung diseases).
- Chronic hepatitis (whether viral or alcohol-induced) leading to cirrhosis 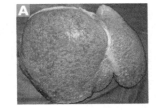 (end-stage liver fibrosis).

Blockage of any hollow organ can lead to infection.

Have you ever heard the saying, "running water never grows stale"? Have you ever left water in a bottle for a few days after drinking from it and notice that it tastes funky when you drink from it again? The point is: stasis allows for bacterial overgrowth.

Some examples of this are:

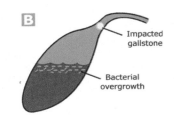
Impacted gallstone

Bacterial overgrowth

- Biliary tract infections (cholecystitis , ascending cholangitis, etc.) caused by a gallstone getting stuck somewhere in the tract.
- Urinary tract infections caused by blockage somewhere in the tract from kidney stones, benign prostatic hyperplasia, tumor, neurogenic bladder, pregnancy, etc.

The suffix "-itis" means inflammation

For example: hepatitis, meningitis and pericarditis.

Having one autoimmune disease predisposes you to having others.

This makes intuitive sense: if your immune system has already mistaken an antigen of yours as foreign, there's a chance it might do it again. Therefore, if a question stem mentions the patient having a history of a certain autoimmune disease and then goes on to talk about some new symptoms, consider the possibility that this might be a new autoimmune disease.

Autoimmune disease is most common in women 20–50.

Autoimmune diseases are 3–4 times more common in women. They generally have an onset between ages 20-50; the *classical* presentation is a woman in her 30s.

- o On exams, if symptoms start after age 50, you should consider an alternative diagnosis. This makes sense because the immune system weakens with advanced age. An exception to this is giant cell arteritis, which usually presents after age 50.

Neoplasia

Metastasis

- The most important hallmark of malignancy is the *potential for metastasis.*
- If you see multiple *cancerous* tumors within an organ, it's almost always metastases 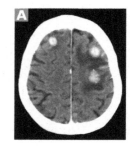 rather than primary tumors.
  - o Think about it: unless there's some extreme predisposition to developing tumors in that organ (e.g., familial adenomatous polyposis), the likelihood of getting hit with multiple new cancers in the same organ within a short time is extremely low. Meanwhile, if cancer cells are being shot into that organ from elsewhere through the blood stream, it absolutely makes sense that you would see multiple discrete tumor foci (e.g., "cannonball lesions").
- Carcinomas usually spread by lymphatics; sarcomas spread through blood.
- The most common sites of metastases relate to venous and lymphatic drainage of the primary site.
  - o Remember: almost all gastrointestinal organs drain to the liver via the portal venous system. It therefore makes sense that malignancy in gastrointestinal organs have a tendency to metastasize to the liver. This includes cancers of the colon, stomach, esophagus, and pancreas.

Cancers generally develop over months.

- If a patient has been complaining of a symptom for a year or more, it's almost certainly NOT cancer.

o   An exception to this is prostate cancer, which is very slow-growing. Most men with prostate cancer die *with* it rather than *from* it.

Less differentiation = more aggressive

Generally, the more undifferentiated (i.e., primitive) a cancer is, the more aggressive it is.

o   This makes sense because primitive cells in general grow and divide very rapidly.

o   It's just like a human: the younger you are, the more rapidly you're growing (proportionally) and hence the more rapidly all of your cells are dividing. As you reach adulthood (i.e., become "differentiated"), you don't need to grow as much.

"-oma" vs. "-carcinoma", "-sarcoma", or "-blastoma".

- Benign tumors end in just "-oma". Malignant tumors tend to end in "-carcinoma", "-sarcoma", or "-blastoma". There are 4 main exceptions where a malignant tumor ends only in "-oma":
  1. Melanoma
  2. Mesothelioma
  3. Leukemia/lymphoma
  4. Seminoma
- Blastomas are small round blue cell cancers that are exquisitely sensitive to radiation therapy.
  o   They're small round blue cells because as the name implies, they're comprised of *blasts* (**precursor cells**). Blast cells in general have large nuclei with lots of DNA, which stains blue on H&E stains.
  o   They're exquisitely sensitive to radiation therapy because of their large nuclei with tons of DNA replication. Remember: radiation damages DNA.
- Adenocarcinomas are carcinomas arising from glandular tissue ("adeno-" means "pertaining to a gland"). Therefore, by definition, they are able to secrete fluid (often mucous).
  o   This mucous/fluid can have clinical implications (e.g., causing pseudomyxoma peritonei – a buildup of gelatinous fluid in the abdomen) and histological importance (e.g., staining mucin positive; signet ring cells [mucin-filled cells] in gastric cancers).

Neurology

- Upper motor neuron (UMN) lesions cause increased tone, hyperreflexia, and no atrophy; lower motor neuron (LMN) lesions cause decreased tone, hyporeflexia, and atrophy.
  o   This makes sense because if there's a lesion in an UMN, a LMN can still fire through other means, and it actually fires abnormally and MORE frequently because the natural inhibitory modulation of UMNs ("descending inhibition") is eliminated. On the other hand, if a LMN is destroyed, the literal trigger for muscle contraction is

eliminated – there's no way around that.

Other

Compensation

Due to compensation, the body can generally cope with *slow* adverse changes much better than *sudden* ones.

- For example, if you're bleeding and your hemoglobin drops from 13g/dL to 9g/dL in a matter of hours, you'll probably be feeling *serious* symptoms. Meanwhile, there are people walking around relatively fine with hemoglobin levels of 5g/dL. This is because their bodies have had time to compensate. The same idea applies to blood pressure.
- Rapid accumulation of pericardial fluid as little as 150mL can severely impede cardiac output (= cardiac tamponade), whereas 1L can accumulate over a longer period without any significant adverse effect!
- COPD patients have a normal oxygen saturation (SpO2) of 88-92%. If a normal person like yourself suddenly dropped to 88-92%, you'd be in serious respiratory distress (normal for healthy people is >95%).

Visceral pain

Visceral (organ) pain is felt at the site of embryologic origin.

- o This is why the pain of getting hit in the gonads for men is felt in the abdomen. The testes originate in the abdomen and later descend into the scrotum. Similarly, the pain of acute cholecystitis and appendicitis start off in the epigastric and umbilical regions, respectively, and only migrate to their actual anatomical locations when the parietal peritoneum (which has *somatic* pain innervation) becomes irritated.

Outpouchings or herniation

Chronically elevated pressure within a walled structure can lead to outpouchings/herniation.

- The 3 major examples of this are:
    - o **Abdominal hernia**: small bowel herniates through the abdominal wall due to persistently increased intraabdominal pressure (e.g., straining from constipation).
    - o **Diverticulosis A**: outpouchings of the descending/sigmoid colon due to persistently increased intraluminal pressure (e.g., straining from constipation).
    - o **Zenker diverticulum B**: excessive pressure in the lower pharynx (from esophageal dysmotility) causes outpouching of the mucosa.
- Elevated pressure in veins doesn't exactly cause outpouchings or herniation, but it does cause dilation, which can cause them to bleed easily. The two most important examples of this are:

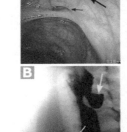

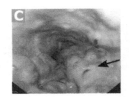

- o **Esophageal varices** 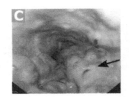 (caused by portal hypertension, usually from liver cirrhosis; can lead to life-threatening hemorrhage)
- o **Hemorrhoids** (caused by constipation and prolonged straining, which increases intraabdominal pressure and causes venous obstruction of rectal veins)

Big 4 imaging tests

The main four imaging tests (in order of lowest to highest resolution):

1. **Ultrasound:** Shows fluid well (appears black), especially when it's against a solid background → hence, shows bladder, gallbladder, pregnant uterus, and abscesses beautifully.
   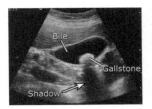
   - o Air is ultrasound's enemy (makes everything fuzzy) → hence, terrible for things like lungs and intestines.
   - o Ultrasound can't penetrate bone → no use for looking at or through bone (e.g., adult's skull).
2. **X-ray:** Based on density. Hence, useful for picking up big *differences* in densities.
   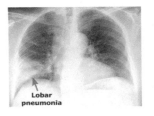
   - o Good for lungs because they should appear quite black due to the air. Abnormal substances stand out as white (e.g. pneumonia, fluid [pleural effusion and pulmonary edema], tumor, etc.)
   - o Good for showing bone fractures.
   - o Decent for bowel obstruction (you see air-fluid levels [fluid pooling at the bottom and air above it]), bowel perforation (you see free air below the diaphragm).
3. **Computerized Tomography (CT):** Essentially a series of x-rays *computerized* together to produce a high-resolution 3D reconstruction. Excellent resolution for pretty much everything. Best imaging test for showing bleeds 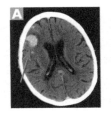. Given that it uses a ton of x-rays, it carries a lot of radiation (e.g. a chest CT has 70x more radiation than a chest X-ray), so it's avoided in pregnancy and young children unless absolutely necessary.
4. **Magnetic Resonance Imaging (MRI):** Uses a *magnetic* field to produce a high-resolution 3D reconstruction. Excellent resolution for pretty much everything. Looks similar to CT, but better for showing soft tissues (e.g., brain, spinal cord, tendons/ligaments, etc.). Since it uses magnets, it carries no radiation (hence it's a good alternative to CT for pregnancy/young children).
   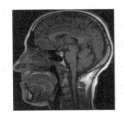

-Ectomy/otomy/ostomy procedures

Procedure	Meaning	Example	Memory Tip
-ectomy	Surgical removal of something	An appendectomy is surgical removal of the appendix	Just think of the word *"resect"*
-otomy	Cutting into something	A craniotomy is a surgery where a hole is made into the brain to relieve pressure A laparotomy is a surgery where an incision is made into the abdominal cavity	Think: -otomy = making a *"dot"* into something
-ostomy	Making a stoma (an alternate pathway in a hollow organ). This can be either putting an artificial tube through the organ (e.g., nephrostomy, tracheostomy) or bringing the organ to the body surface to drain (e.g. colostomy)	A nephrostomy is a draining tube placed into the kidney (renal pelvis) to allow for urine drainage when there's an obstruction in the ureter A colostomy is a surgery where one portion of the colon is brought to the abdominal wall surface to allow poop to empty into a bag (a stoma)	Think: make a stoma to *"store"* (or *"stow"* away) the organ's contents elsewhere

Laparotomy

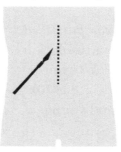

Appendectomy

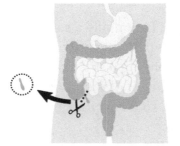

Colostomy

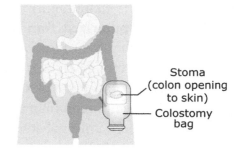

Stoma (colon opening to skin)

Colostomy bag

> **Tips & key concepts: Pathognomonic features**

For the purposes of basic science exams, consider the following findings as pathognomonic for the corresponding disease. These are really valuable to know because as soon as you see the given feature in the question stem, the diagnosis is done.

Cardiovascular

- Aschoff bodies 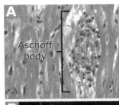 → Rheumatic heart disease
    - Aschoff bodies are granulomas with giant cells in the heart.
- Machine-like heart murmur → Patent ductus arteriosus
- Pericardial friction rub → Pericarditis
- Pulsatile abdominal mass → Abdominal aortic aneurysm
- Boot-shaped heart on chest X-ray 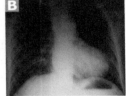 → Tetralogy of Fallot
    - Think: If you want to **Fallot** (follow) someone, you need to put on your **boots**.
- Cyanosis improved by squatting → Tetralogy of Fallot
    - Squatting increases systemic vascular resistance → higher pressure in left heart → less right-to-left shunting → more blood reaches lungs.
- "String of beads" artery → Fibromuscular dysplasia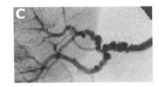
    - Most commonly in the renal arteries (→ causes hypertension).
    - It makes sense why this disease produces arteries that look like this: as the name implies, there are on-and-off deposits of *fibrous tissue* along an artery, causing constrictions at intervals.
- Delta wave 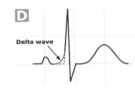 on ECG → Wolff-Parkinson-White syndrome
    - A delta wave is a slurring of the upstroke at the start of the QRS complex.
    - Think: A **wolf** scares your heart into starting its depolarization early.

Endocrine

- Trousseau and Chvostek signs → Hypocalcemia
    - **Trousseau sign:** contraction of hand/wrist when blood pressure cuff is inflated.
        - **Trousseau** → cuff around the **Triceps**
    - **Chvostek sign:** contraction of facial muscles when area of facial nerve is tapped.
        - **Chvostek** → tapping the **Cheek**
- Buffalo hump → Cushing syndrome
- Bilateral exophthalmos (bulging eyes) → Graves' disease

Gastrointestinal

- Kayser-Fleischer rings **A** → Wilson's disease
  - Kayser-Fleischer rings are brown rings of copper deposition on the cornea that encircle the iris.
- Rice-water stools → Cholera
- Olive-shaped abdominal mass in a child → Pyloric stenosis
- Pneumatosis intestinalis **B** in newborn (gas in bowel wall) → Necrotizing enterocolitis
- Murphy's sign → Acute cholecystitis
  - Murphy's sign: a halt in inspiration when you suddenly palpate the liver edge.

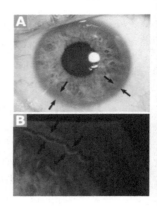

Hematology

- Reed-Sternberg ("Owl-eye") cells **A** → Hodgkin Lymphoma
  - These are *cells* that have an owl's eye appearance - don't confuse this with the owl eye *inclusion bodies* of cytomegalovirus infection.
- Auer rods **B** → Acute myeloid leukemia
  - Auer rods are pink, needle-shaped cytoplasmic inclusion bodies.
  - Think: one **Auer** (hour) is an **AML** (ample) amount of time.
- Howell-Jolly bodies **C** → Asplenia/hyposplenia
  - Howell-Jolly bodies are basophilic nuclear remnants inside RBCs that are normally removed by splenic macrophages.
  - Think: you get **Howell**-Jolly bodies if your spleen is **hollow**. This causes your RBCs to actually be NOT hollow.
- Heinz bodies and bite cells → G6PD deficiency
  - Think: take a **bite** of your burger with **Heinz** ketchup (G6PD kind of sounds like a type of burger, doesn't it? The ol' G-6 PounDer).
- Neoplasm with "tennis-racket" organelles (Birbeck granules **D**) → Langerhans Cell Histiocytosis
  - I bet having **longer hands** (Langerhans) makes you a better **tennis** player.

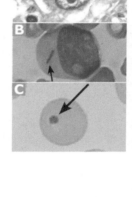

Infections

- "Owl eye" inclusion bodies → Cytomegalovirus
  - These are *intracellular* *inclusion bodies* (makes sense, as viruses enter inside cells) - don't confuse them with the Reed-Sternberg (Owl eye) *cells* of Hodgkin Lymphoma.
- Bull's-eye rash (erythema migrans) → Lyme disease
  - Picture throwing a lime right through the bullseye of a target.
- Risus sardonicus → Tetanus

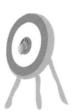

- Risus sardonicus is the sustained spasm of facial muscles, which appears to produce grinning.
- Koplik spots 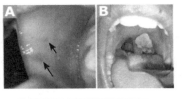 → Measles
  - Koplik spots are clustered, bluish-white spots on the buccal mucosa.
- Pseudomembrane **B** on tonsils/pharynx → Diphtheria
- Hydrophobia and Negri bodies → Rabies
  - Negri bodies are eosinophilic inclusion bodies in the cytoplasm of pyramidal cells of the hippocampus (think: *hippos* (hippocampus) are not one of the animals that can give you rabies but it would be slightly comedic if they could).
- Kernig's and Brudzinski's signs → Meningitis
  - Brudzinski's sign: flexion of neck causes involuntary flexion of hips and knees.
  - Kernig's sign: inability to straighten knee when hips are flexed to 90 degrees (think: "**K**" for **K**nee).
- Maltese cross in RBCs **C** → Babesiosis
- Leonine facies → Leprosy
- Hutchinson teeth **D** and Mulberry molars → Congenital syphilis
- Strawberry cervix → Trichomoniasis
  - Nobody wanna see this kind of *strawberry trick…*

> **! TIP**
>
> Search "rabies patient" on YouTube. You probably won't forget rabies' association with hydrophobia after what you see…

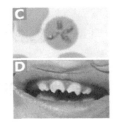

Musculoskeletal and Dermatology

- Bamboo spine **A** on X-ray → Ankylosing spondylitis
- Tophi → Gout
  - Tophi are deposits of monosodium urate in joints.
- Calf pseudohypertrophy → Muscular dystrophy (e.g., Duchenne)
- Heberden nodes **B** (DIP joint swelling) → Osteoarthritis
  - Rheumatoid arthritis DOES NOT affect distal interphalangeal (DIP) joints.
  - Think: after a lifetime of hard work and wear and tear (*i.e., osteoarthritis*), it's time to go for **dips** in the pool.
- Wickham striae **C** → Lichen planus
  - Wickham striae are white lines, typically in the oral mucosa.
  - Think of it as "**White**ham striae", and then remember how **planes** (planus) leave those *white lines* in the sky.
- "Christmas tree" rash → Pityriasis rosea
  - Think: if a person went out to get a Christmas tree and instead came home with this rash, you can imagine their family would think that's a real **pity** (*pityriasis*). Probably not the Christmas tree they were expecting.

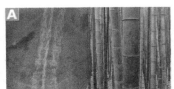

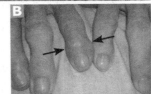

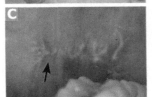

- Silvery scaling plaques on skin → Psoriasis **A**
  - Think: **Psorry**, this **silver** isn't actually worth anything.
- "Stuck-on", greasy skin lesion → Seborrheic keratosis **B**
  - It makes sense that it appears "stuck-on": as the name implies, it's a large pile of _keratinocytes_, which are found only in the epidermis – the outermost layer of the skin.
- Crusted, honey-coloured skin lesion → Impetigo **C**
  - Think: A lesion this delicious-sounding would make anyone **impatient** (_impetigo_) (it looks like _honey_ and it even has _crust!_ Yum!)
- Dark, thick skin patches in armpits → Acanthosis nigricans **D**
  - In Latin, _"Nigricans"_ means _"blackening"_, so just think about the name.
  - Remember that acanthosis nigricans is associated with insulin resistance (e.g., diabetes, PCOS) and gastric cancer.

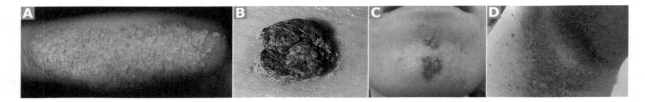

Neurology

- Pill-rolling tremor → Parkinson's disease
- Bilateral internuclear ophthalmoplegia → Multiple sclerosis
  - Conjugate horizontal gaze impairment due to medial longitudinal fasciculus (MLF) lesion.
- Bilateral acoustic schwannomas → Neurofibromatosis type 2
  - "**2** acoustic schwannomas is NF **2**".
- Excruciating brief headache with lacrimation → Cluster headache
- 14-3-3 protein in CSF → Creutzfeldt-Jakob disease
  - Think of Creutzfeldt-Jakob disease as the disease with way too many letters and numbers. The name itself has like 10 letters that don't need to be there, and then you have this 14-3-3 stuff going on. Whoever's naming this stuff needs to settle down.

Renal

- Muddy brown casts → Acute tubular necrosis
  - Makes sense – cells turn brown and look dirty when they die off.
- Waxy casts → Chronic renal failure/end-stage renal disease
  - Think of _wax_ sculptures, which are lifeless versions of whatever they're sculpted after. Similarly, think of waxy casts as signifying a lifeless kidney (i.e., ESRD).

Reproductive

- Call-Exner bodies **A** → Granulosa cell tumor
  - Call-Exner bodies are follicle-like granulosa cells arranged haphazardly around collections of eosinophilic fluid.
- Schiller-Duval bodies **B** → Yolk sac tumor
  - Schiller-Duval bodies are blood vessels surrounded by tumor, which make them look like glomeruli.
  - I always pictured Schiller-Duval bodies as **Shelly Duvall** – the actress who played Mrs. Torrance in the movie The Shining. (Spoiler Alert) Instead of Jack trying to kill her with an ax, I'd picture him throwing **eggs** (think: egg **yolk**) at her. This murderous scene also helped me remember that Schiller-Duval bodies are **blood** vessels.
- Reinke crystals → Leydig cell tumor
  - Think: "Some guys like to **rank** (Reinke) the **ladies** (Leydig)" (this makes even more sense given this is a testicular tumor…).
- "Snowstorm" or "cluster of grapes" uterus **C** on ultrasound → Complete hydatidiform mole
- Blue-domed breast cysts→ Fibrocystic changes

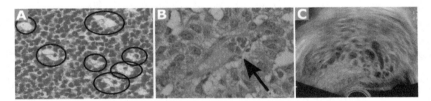

Respiratory

- Barrel-chest **D** → COPD
- Pleural plaques **E** → Asbestosis

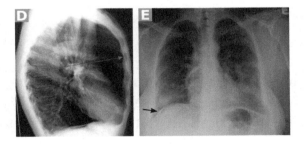

Other

- Cat's (white) eye reflex → Retinoblastoma
- Raccoon eyes + Battle sign → Basilar skull fracture
  - Raccoon eyes: periorbital ecchymosis
  - Battle sign: mastoid ecchymosis

> **Tips & key concepts: Specific tricks & mnemonics**

The following are more specific tips and mnemonics. Read these around the time you're studying that particular organ system.

Cardiovascular

Dressler syndrome

Autoimmune pericarditis after a myocardial infarction.

- o Think: **Dress**ler syndrome is when the heart sheds its "**dress**" after an infarction (i.e., releasing new antigens the body has never seen before), leading to an autoimmune attack against these newly-encountered antigens.

Turner syndrome

- Coarctation of the aorta is associated with **Turner** syndrome.
  - o Think: in coarctation of the aorta, the aorta becomes narrowed right after it **Turns** the corner (i.e., right after the aortic arch)
- Turner syndrome is also associated with a bicuspid aortic valve.
  - o Think: just like they're missing an X chromosome, they might also be missing an aortic valve.

Bacterial endocarditis

Osler nodes vs. Janeway lesions: both are signs of bacterial endocarditis, but Osler nodes are tender and on finger/toe pads, while Janeway lesions are painless and on palms/soles.

- o Think: **O**uch, **O**sler!

Acute pericarditis

Acute pericarditis causes diffuse ST-segment elevation and PR depression.

- o Think: Pe**R**icarditis → **PR** depression

Kussmaul sign

Kussmaul sign is a paradoxical increase in jugular venous pressure (JVP) 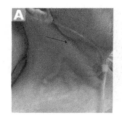 on inspiration instead of the normal decrease. It's caused by impaired filling of the right ventricle (e.g., constrictive pericarditis, restrictive cardiomyopathies).

- o Think: when you're angry and **cuss**ing *(Kussmaul)*, your jugular vein pops out.

Giant cell (temporal) arteritis

The feared complication of giant cell (temporal) arteritis is blindness.

o   Think: the temporal artery runs right beside the eye, so it makes sense that temporal arteritis can affect vision.

Kawasaki disease

Kawasaki disease causes conjunctival injection, rash, oral mucositis (strawberry tongue), hand-foot edema/erythema, and coronary artery aneurysms.

o   Picture a little kid riding a **Kawasaki** motorcycle really fast. The intense wind causes irritation and makes his **eyes**, **skin**, and **tongue** turn red. His **hands** and **feet** are also getting swollen from gripping the bike so intensely. He's having so much excitement that he might have a **heart attack** (coronary artery aneurysm)!

Churg-Strauss syndrome

The most common sign of Churg-**Strauss** syndrome (eosinophilic granulomatosis with polyangiitis) is adult-onset asthma.

o   Think: They say asthma is like breathing through a **straw**.

Polyarteritis nodosa

Polyarteritis nodosa has an association with Hepatitis B.

o   Think: Hepatitis causes nodes in your liver (cirrhosis) and nodes in your arteries (polyarteritis nodosa).

Endocrine

Cushing syndrome vs. Cushing disease

A syndrome is a group of signs/symptoms that occur together, while a disease is something that has a clearly defined cause. Therefore, it makes sense that Cushing syndrome is simply symptoms from high cortisol. Cushing disease, on the other hand, is an ACTH-secreting pituitary adenoma and is *one cause* of Cushing syndrome.

Riedel thyroiditis

Thyroid replaced by **fibrous** tissue (sometimes becomes "hard as **wood**").

o   Think: A **reed** is a tall, **fibrous** grass, and also a thin strip of **wood** in musical instruments (if unfamiliar, look these up in Google Images).

Multiple endocrine neoplasias

Multiple endocrine neoplasias (MEN syndromes): progressively contain more "M's".

- MEN 1: **PPP** (**P**ituitary adenoma, **P**ancreatic endocrine tumors, **P**arathyroid adenomas).
- MEN 2A: **PPM** (**P**arathyroid hyperplasia, **P**heochromocytoma, **M**edullary thyroid carcinoma).

- MEN 2B: **PMM** (**P**heochromocytoma, **M**edullary thyroid carcinoma, **M**ucosal neuromas).

Thyroid carcinoma

- **Follicular** thyroid carcinoma is associated with **RAS** mutation.
  - <u>Think</u>: **RAS**pberries are good for your **follicles** (not sure if they really are though…)
- **Papillary** thyroid carcinoma is associated with **BRAF** (and RET) mutation.
  - <u>Think</u>: **Papi** makes you **barf**

Gastrointestinal

Boerhaave syndrome vs. Mallory-Weiss tear

- Boerhaave syndrome is a *transmural* perforation of the esophagus.
  - <u>Think</u>: **Boer**haave syndrome **bores** a hole through the esophagus.
- Mallory-Weiss tear is a *partial-thickness* mucosal laceration of the esophagus.
  - <u>Think</u>: Mallory is a female name, and hence Mallory-Weiss tear is the gentler one (alternatively, just remember Boerhaave and think of Mallory-Weiss as "the other one").

Plummer-Vinson syndrome

Plummer-Vinson syndrome: triad of esophageal webs, dysphagia, and iron deficiency anemia.

  - <u>Think</u>: in **Plummer**-Vinson syndrome, you need a **Plumber** to unclog the blockage (dysphagia) caused by the esophageal webs.

Ménétrier disease

Ménétrier disease: hyperplasia of gastric mucosa → hypertrophied rugae

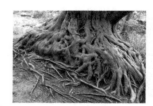

  - <u>Think</u>: in **Ménétrier** disease, your gastric mucosa looks like the roots of a **tree**.

Hirschsprung disease

Hirschsprung disease: lack of ganglion cells/enteric nervous plexuses in distal colon → defective relaxation/peristalsis in that segment → congenital megacolon and obstruction. Increased risk in Down syndrome.

  - <u>Think</u>: in Hirsch**sprung**, a segment of bowel loses its **spring** (i.e., peristalsis). **Down** syndrome babies may have trouble getting their poop **down**.

Crohn disease

Remember **Crohn** disease by thinking of a **crown** (see picture).

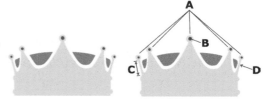

- A → Skip lesions
- B → Noncaseating granulomas (represented by the jewels within the little round thingies)
- C → Transmural inflammation
- D → Fistulas

Hepatic adenomas

Hepatic adenomas are often related to oral contraceptive use.

- Girl: should I take oral contraceptives?
- Liver: "*I don't know man…*" *(adenoma)*

Dubin-Johnson syndrome

Dubin-Johnson syndrome: grossly black liver

> o Think: in **Dubin**-Johnson syndrome, the liver turns grossly black, so you need to throw it into **da bin**.

Hematology

Lymphoma vs. leukemia

- **Lymph**oma is a discrete tumor mass arising from within a **lymph** node. It's comprised of **lymph**ocytes.
- **Leuk**emia is a cancerous proliferation of **leuk**ocytes (myeloid or lymphoid) starting in the bone barrow (because that's where leukocytes are produced), with the cancerous cells traveling all throughout the blood stream (again, just like leukocytes!)

Hodgkin vs. non-Hodgkin lymphoma

- **Hodgkin:** since it has the characteristic "*owl* cells" (Reed-Sternberg cells), picture Hodgkin lymphoma as a gentle *owl*. An owl stays close to its nest – hence, Hodgkin lymphoma is localized to a **single group of nodes** (= makes sense that it has **better prognosis**) and has **contiguous spread** (spread to *adjacent* rather than distant nodes). Again, since it has the better prognosis, it makes sense it's also associated with the less sinister virus – **EBV** (vs. HIV in non-Hodgkin lymphoma).
- **Non-Hodgkin:** simply think of the opposite of Hodgkin characteristics (multiple nodes, extranodal involvement, noncontiguous spread, worse prognosis, and HIV association). (Additionally, you can think: **non**-Hodgkin → **non**contiguous spread).

Non-Hodgkin lymphoma translocations

Memorize the translocations by remembering the *difference* between the two numbers. This way, you only have to remember one number for each lymphoma subtype. For example, Burkitt lymphoma has a translocation between chromosomes 8 and 14, making the difference 6. Each lymphoma subtype has a unique number, so you don't have to worry about mixing them up.

- **Mantle** cell lymphoma: **3** (t[11;14])
  - Mickey **Mantle** was a great baseball player (make the "*OK sign*" with 3 fingers).
- Follicular lymphoma: **4** (t[14;18])
  - Either pronounce it "**Four**-icular" or picture **four**-leaf clovers growing out of all your hair follicles.
- Burkitt lymphoma: **6** (t[8;14])
  - People often play **dice** (*symbolizes* 6) by throwing it out of a cup, which is basically like a little **bucket** (*Burkitt*).
- Marginal zone lymphoma: **7** (t[11;18])
  - Think about having a **one-week** (i.e., 7 days) **margin** between classes or semesters. Alternatively, think "keep a great **margin** between you and the 7 deadly sins".

Leukemia mnemonics

- **ALL:** usually in children
  - Think: **ALL** affects **all** ages (i.e., children too; other leukemias usually just in adults/elderly).
- **CLL:** **smudge** cells
  - Think of **CLL** as a phone **call**. When you dial a number on your cellphone to call someone, you inevitably **smudge** the screen.
- **Hairy cell leukemia:** marrow fibrosis → dry tap on aspiration; pancytopenia; stains TRAP+
  - It makes sense that having tons of fuzzy/hairy cells in the marrow causes fuzzy/fibrotic marrow. If all of your marrow is fibrotic, obviously you can't produce any kind of blood cell (= pancytopenia).
  - Think: all those fuzzy, hair-like projections **TRAP** things well (= **TRAP**+ stain).
- **AML:** Auer rods
  - An **Auer** (hour) is an **AMPLE** (**AML**) amount of time.
- **CML:** Philadelphia chromosome (t[9;22], BRC-ABL); very low LAP (vs. high in leukemoid reaction).
  - Think of **CML** as a **camel**. If you ever were to let a camel loose in a crowded city like **Philadelphia**, it would break everything that's **breakable** (**BRC-ABL**) and you'd have to call **9-2-2** (think: the more serious version of 9-1-1).
  - LAP is an enzyme in the granules of granulocytes. Since the granulocytes in CML are cancerous and abnormal, it makes sense that this enzyme would be low compared to properly functioning granulocytes in a leukemoid reaction.

Heme synthesis conditions

1. **Acute intermittent porphyria:** defective porphobilinogen deaminase. Psychiatric disturbances.
    o   <u>Think</u>: sometimes, women get **acute, intermittent DMs** (**DE-AM**-inase) from creepy guys and it drives them **crazy** (psychiatric disturbances).
2. **Porphyria cutanea tarda:** defective uroporphyrinogen decarboxylase. Blistering cutaneous photosensitivity and hyperpigmentation.
    o   **"Cutanea"** literally tells you it has **cutaneous** (skin) manifestations.
    o   You know what else irritates the skin? **Urine**. Let that remind you of **uro**porphyrinogen decarboxylase.
3. **Lead poisoning:** inhibits ferrochelatase and ALAD. Neurologic/psychiatric symptoms.
    o   Lead is a metal, and it inhibits the enzyme with a metal in its name ('ferro-' = iron). **ALAD** also sounds/looks like **LEAD**.
    o   Lead is a metal, and metals conduct electricity (reminds you of neurologic symptoms).

Musculoskeletal & Skin

Strawberry vs. cherry hemangiomas

Strawberry hemangiomas are seen in infants, while cherry hemangiomas are seen in the elderly.

   o   <u>Think</u>: **infants** can pick **strawberries** (because they grow at ground level), but you have to be an **adult** to pick **cherries** (they grow high up in trees).

Sjögren syndrome

Think of this as "that Scandinavian syndrome" (Sjögren is a Swedish name). Picture a Scandinavian woman getting her lacrimal and salivary glands dried out by the extreme Scandinavian cold (= exocrine gland destruction and resulting corneal, parotid and dental damage). You can even picture her drinking a malt beverage to remember Sjögren syndrome can lead to MALToma development.

Systemic lupus erythematosus

Systemic lupus erythematosus antibodies:

- **ANA:** sensitive but not at all specific.
    o   Read **ANA** as "*ANY*" → it can be elevated in almost *ANY* autoimmune condition (or at least many others).
- **Anti-Smith antibodies:** specific
    o   "Smith" is a *specific* person's name.
- **Antihistone antibodies:** sensitive for **drug**-induced lupus
    o   "Antihistone" sounds just like "antihistamine" – a **drug** (alternative: "*hi-stoned on drugs*")

Polymyositis vs. dermatomyositis

- **Polymyositis:** endomysial inflammation
- **Dermatomyositis:** perimysial inflammation
  - It makes sense that the condition with skin involvement (**dermato**myositis) is the one that inflames the more superficial layer (perimysium) i.e., the layer closer to the skin.

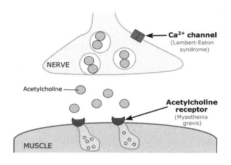

Neuromuscular junction diseases

- **Lambert-Eaton myasthenic syndrome:** autoantibodies to presynaptic Ca^{2+} channel
  - Lambert-**Eaton** deals with the one that you can **eat** (calcium, e.g., milk).
- **Myasthenia gravis:** autoantibodies to postsynaptic ACh receptor
  - 'The other one'.

Pemphigus vulgaris vs. bullous pemphigoid

- Pemphigus **vulgaris** involves the **oral mucosa**, while bullous pemphigoid doesn't.
  - <u>Think</u>: **vulgar** words are spoken from the **mouth**.
  - Additionally, remember that bullous pemphigoid is the less severe one while pemphigus vulgaris is potentially fatal by thinking of the suffix *"-oid"* in bullous *pemphigoid*. This means it's *"kind of like"* pemphigus vulgaris but it doesn't quite match up. Pemphigus vulgaris' name is original – it's the real deal.

Skin pigment disorders

- **Vitiligo:** irregular areas of complete depigmentation caused by autoimmune destruction of melanocytes.
  - **Vitiligo** sounds like *"wait 'til I go"*. Use this to remind you that in vitiligo, your melanocytes (and your skin pigment) *go*.
- **Melasma:** hyperpigmentation (increased **mela**nin production) associated with pregnancy ("mask of pregnancy") or OCP use.

Neurology

Decorticate vs. decerebrate posturing

Decorticate posturing has arm flexion (patient brings arms to their **core**), while decerebrate posturing has arm extension.

Decorticate

Decerebrate

- Remember that decerebrate is the worse one by thinking that in decorticate posturing, the patient is at least making an effort to protect themself by drawing their arms in, while in decerebrate posturing it's as though they've given up.

- o Note: the actual reasoning is that decerebrate posturing indicates brainstem damage [red nucleus], while in de**corticate** posturing the brainstem is spared [i.e., just **cortical** damage].

Bilateral paralysis from stroke

Remember that amongst the major brain and brainstem stroke syndromes, a basilar artery stroke is the only one that always produces BILATERAL paralysis throughout the body (= **locked-in syndrome**). This is because there is only one basilar artery, while the other major arteries have left and right branches.

Transtentorial vs. uncal herniation

- **Transtentorial herniation:** central/downward herniation of brain
  - o <u>Think</u> of a **tent** collapsing straight down on you. Just look at an image of the tentorium cerebelli and this will make sense (the tentorium cerebelli is what separates the brain from the brainstem). Remember that transtentorial herniation can rupture the paramedian basilar artery branches because the basilar artery is centrally located (straight along the pons).
- **Uncal herniation:** subtype of transtentorial herniation where the uncus (medial temporal lobe) herniates through the tentorium cerebelli.
  - o <u>Think</u>: **Uncal** herniation is just like an **uncle**: you're not a straight-down descendant of his – it goes sideways and down (i.e., you're his sibling's child). Also, picture not being able to look your **uncle** in the eye to remember that uncal herniation causes "down-and-out" gaze via compression of the ipsilateral CN 3.

Causes of a cherry-red spot on the macula

Cherry Trees Never Grow Tall

1. Central retinal artery occlusion
2. Tay-Sachs disease
3. Niemann-Pick disease
4. Gaucher disease
5. Trauma (Berlin's edema)

Craniopharyngiomas

Craniopharyngiomas are tumors derived from remnants of Rathke pouch that grow near the pituitary gland. They often have calcifications and cholesterol crystals.

- o <u>Think</u> of a **rat pit** (Rathke – pituitary) where the rats are feasting on **milk** (**calcium**) and chips (or some high **cholesterol** food).

Oncology

Bcl-2 and Bcl-x vs. BAX and BAK

Bcl-2 and Bcl-x are antiapoptotic (prevent cell death), while BAX and BAK are proapoptotic (induce cell death). Malignancy can result from both overexpression of antiapoptotic proteins and underproduced/defective proapoptotic proteins.

- o **Bcl** stands for *B-cell lymphoma*. As its name implies, this protein plays a role in B-cell lymphoma development (amongst other cancers) by preventing apoptosis. Therefore, simply think about the name.
- o **BAX** and **BAK**: Think "**Back**space", just like the key on your keyboard. When you make a mistake, you press Backspace to delete it.

Hamartomas

Hamartomas are benign growths made up of an **abnormal mixture of cells and tissues** native to the area in which it grows.

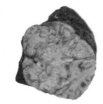

- o Think of a **hamar**toma as a **hammer**, which can be used to craft **many different types of items**.

Keratin pearls

Keratin pearls 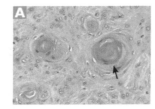 are often seen in squamous cell carcinomas.

- o This makes sense because as you learned in histology, **keratin** often forms the apical layer of stratified **squamous** epithelium (e.g., skin).

Renal

Electrolyte derangements

For exam purposes, follow this simplification to score some easy points:

- If the main problem is **arrhythmia**, the derangement is probably **potassium**.
- If the main problem is in the **brain** (e.g., coma, confusion), the derangement is probably **sodium** (or glucose).
- If the main problem is in the **muscles** (e.g., muscle spasms/twitching, tetany), the derangement is probably **calcium**.

Renal tubular defects

- Fanconi syndrome: **proximal** tubule
    - o Think: when it's hot, you want to bring the **fan** more **proximal** to you.
- **Bar**ter syndrome: loop of Henle
    - o Think: **Bart** Simpson → loop of Homer.

- **Gitelman** syndrome: **distal** tubule
  - Think: A true **gentleman** keeps his **distance** from the ladies.
- **Liddle** syndrome: collecting duct
  - Think: Just a **liddle** more to go! (i.e., it's the last part of the nephron).

Alport syndrome

Mutation in type 4 collagen → splitting of glomerular basement membrane (basket-weave appearance); eye problems and sensorineural deafness.

  - Picture a scene at an **airport** (*"Alport"*). A passenger is getting off the plane with his flimsy **basket-weave** bag made of **collagen**, and the **bottom is splitting open**. The passenger's **eyes** and **ears** are getting damaged by the super loud plane sounds and the wind from the engine.

Kidney stone shapes

- Calcium **oxalate** : **envelope** or dumbbell
  - Think: Perhaps in the past they used **ox**en to deliver mail/ **envelopes**?
- Magnesium ammonium phosphate (**MAP**) : **coffin** lid
  - Think: Treasure **maps** often lead to tombs (**coffins**).
- Cystine : hexagonal
  - Think: Drop the "1" in **16** (*cystine*) and you get **6** (*i.e., hexagon*).

UTI vs. pyelonephritis

It's really important – *both* for exams and real life – to know that systemic symptoms like fever and chills are generally **absent** in simple urinary tract infections (acute bacterial cystitis). If they *are* present, it tells you the infection has likely ascended to the kidneys (= pyelonephritis). This makes sense – the bladder is like a sealed chamber, and so infection mainly just irritates the inner wall. The kidneys, on the other hand, are highly perfused (think of the nephron) and hence its infection will increase inflammatory mediators all throughout the systemic circulation.

Reproductive

Teratomas

Teratomas 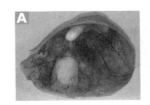 are tumors (often of the ovary) containing elements from more than one primitive germ cell layer. Mature teratomas can have tissue like hair, teeth, skin, and bone (scary, right?) Hence, whenever you hear "**teratoma**", think "*terafying*".

Asherman syndrome

Asherman syndrome is when something scars the endometrium – usually a procedure like dilation and curettage (scraping) – leading to amenorrhea and infertility.

- o Think: **Asherman** syndrome is when the endometrium is turned into **ash**.

Bloody nipple discharge

Remember the 3 causes of bloody nipple discharge: intraductal papilloma, duct ectasia, and breast cancer.

Phyllodes tumor

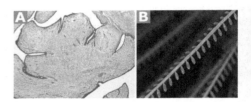

Phyllodes tumor 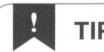 is a large mass with leaf-like lobulations.

- o A "**phyllode**" B is actually a plant **leaf** stem. If you need help remembering that, the "*phyll-*" should remind you of chloro**phyll**. Additionally, picture a really big leaf to remember Phyllodes tumors are large.

Paget disease

A breast cancer that causes eczematous **patches** on the nipple.

Prehn's sign

Prehn's sign: elevation of testicle relieves pain. A positive sign points towards epididymitis, while a negative sign to testicular torsion.

- o Think: the testes are hanging and pulling down on the spermatic cord, stretching it. If the epididymis is inflamed, this stretching will hurt, and hence elevating the scrotum will provide some relief. On the other hand, elevating the testicle isn't going to untangle twisted blood vessels in torsion.

> **! TIP**
>
> For real-life clinical practice, Prehn's sign has been shown to be **unreliable** in distinguishing torsion from epididymitis. **Absent cremasteric reflex** is actually the most accurate clinical sign of testicular torsion.

Respiratory

Asbestosis

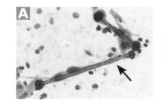

Asbestosis causes formation of asbestos bodies 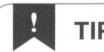 (iron-rich bodies that resemble dumbbells); affects lower lobes of lungs.

- o Think: iron dumbbells are heavy, and hence it makes sense that asbestosis is the only pneumoconiosis that affects the *lower* lobes of the lungs.
- o Remember: Prussian blue stains highlight iron deposition, hence they can identify asbestos bodies ("**Russians** like to pump **iron!**")

Squamous and Small cell carcinomas

Squamous and **S**mall cell carcinomas of the lung are often associated with **S**moking and are **S**entral (central) in location.

Small cell carcinoma

Small cell carcinoma might be small but it packs a big punch through its paraneoplastic syndromes:

- Cushing syndrome
- SIADH
- Lambert-Eaton syndrome
- Encephalitis/subacute cerebellar degeneration

Lung adenocarcinoma

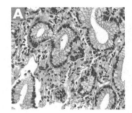

Think of lung adenocarcinoma as the "wild animal" cancer. Activating mutations include **EGFR**, **ALK**, and **KRAS**, so picture a **giraffe** and an **elk** eating **grass** near their **den** (adenocarcinoma).

- o Remember: it's an adenocarcinoma (carcinoma of glandular tissue). It therefore makes sense that on histology, it will have a glandular pattern 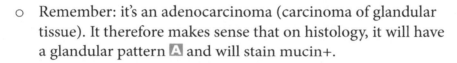 and will stain mucin+.

Image Credits

Index

Made in the USA
Columbia, SC
14 April 2022

58988895R00117